# Introductory
# laboratory exercises
# for medical technologists

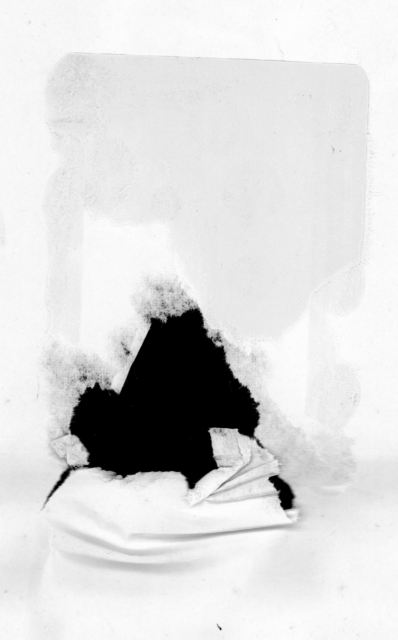

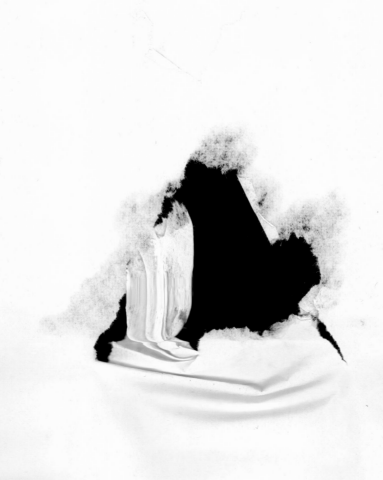

# Preface

This manual is an outgrowth of a one-semester course that has been given for several years to students in medical technology at Brigham Young University. The course was designed to introduce the students to the field of medical technology by performing simple clinical laboratory procedures. Brief explanations of test principles are given so that the student may appreciate the indications for such procedures. The material in the manual may be supplemented in class by photomicrographs and demonstration materials to provide a more graphic understanding of the laboratory procedures.

The manual should be considered as an introduction to laboratory procedures and not as a complete presentation of the subject. Upon completion of the course, the student will have had adequate exposure with laboratory procedures so that he or she will be able to make a rational decision concerning a career in laboratory medicine.

I would like to thank all my students for inspiring the book and my mother for typing the manuscript.

Shauna C. Anderson

v

# Contents

# Introductory laboratory exercises for medical technologists

# 1 Medical terminology

The following work elements are commonly used to construct medical terms

| Element | Definition | Element | Definition |
|---|---|---|---|
| a- | absent or deficient | dis- | apart, away from |
| ab- | away from | duct- | lead, conduct |
| abdomin- | abdomen | dur- | hard |
| ac- | to (*see* af-) | dys- | bad, improper |
| acou- | hear | e- | out, from |
| af- | to | ect- | outside, without |
| a-, an- | without, not | -ectomize | to subject to excision |
| ant(i)-, | signifying against | -ectomy | excision of organ or part |
| ante- | before in time or place | ede- | swell |
| arthr- | joint | end(o)- | inside |
| auto- | self | enter(o)- | intestine |
| bi- | two | epi- | upon, after, in addition |
| bio- | life | | |
| brachi- | arm | erythro- | red |
| brachy- | short | ex- | out of |
| brady- | slow | extra- | outside of, beyond, in addition |
| cac- | bad, ill | | |
| calc- | stone | fasci- | band |
| capit- | head | febr- | fever |
| carcin- | cancer | -ferent | bear, carry |
| cardi- | heart | fiss- | split |
| caud- | tail | for- | opening |
| cephal- | head | gastr(o)- | stomach |
| chol- | bile | gloss- | tongue |
| chro- | color | gran- | grain, particle |
| cis- | cut, kill | grav- | heavy |
| corp- | body | hem(at)- | blood |
| cyan- | blue | hemi- | half |
| de- | down, from | hepat(o)- | liver |
| derm- | skin | hetero- | the other |
| di- | two | hist(o)-, hist(io)- | web, tissue |
| dipl- | double | | |

| Element | Definition | Element | Definition |
|---------|------------|---------|------------|
| hydro- | water | orth- | straight, right, normal |
| hyper- | above, beyond, extreme | oss- | bone |
| hypo- | under, below | ot(o)- | ear |
| -ia | state or condition | par- | give birth to, bear |
| idi- | peculiar, separate, distinct | para- | beside, beyond |
| infra- | beneath | path- | that which undergoes sickness |
| inter- | among, between | pen- | need, lack |
| intra- | inside | per- | through |
| -ion | process | peri- | around |
| -itis | denoting inflammation | phil- | have an affinity for |
| junct- | yoke, join | phleb(o)- | vein |
| labi- | lip | phob- | fear, dread |
| later- | side | pne- | breathing |
| leuk- | white | pod- | foot |
| lip- | fat | poly- | much, many |
| -logy | science of | post- | after, behind in time or place |
| lute- | yellow | pre- | before in time or place |
| ly- | loose, dissolve | pro- | before in time or place |
| macr- | large, long | pseudo- | false |
| mal- | bad, abnormal | py(o)- | pus |
| medi- | middle | re- | back |
| mega- | great, large | ren(o)- | kidney |
| melan- | black | retro- | backwards |
| mes- | middle | -rrhage | excessive flow |
| micr(o)- | small | -rrhea | flow or discharge |
| mon(o)- | one, single | sanguin- | blood |
| morph(o)- | form, shape | sarc- | flesh |
| multi- | many, much | -sect | cut |
| my(o)- | muscle | -sis | state or condition |
| narc- | numbness, stupor | -stalsis | contraction |
| ne(o)- | new, young | sub- | under, below |
| necr(o)- | corpse, dead | super- | above, addition, implying excess |
| nephr(o)- | kidney | supra- | above, upper, over |
| neur(o)- | nerve | syn- | with, together |
| ob- | against, toward, in front of | tac- | order, arrange |
| oc- | against | tachy- | swift, rapid |
| -odyn- | pain | tens- | stretch |
| -oid | resembling | tetra- | four |
| olig- | few, small | therm- | heat |
| -oma | tumor | thorac- | chest |
| oo- | egg | thromb(o)- | lump, clot |
| or- | mouth | | |
| orchi- | testicles | | |

| Element | Definition | Element | Definition |
|---------|-----------|---------|-----------|
| tom(y)- | cut | ur(o)- | urine, urinary organs or tract |
| tox- | poison | vas- | vessel |
| tract- | draw, drag | vit- | life |
| tri- | three | zyg(o)- | union, join |
| uni- | one | | |

*See worksheets, pp. 73-75.*

# 2 Hematology

**COLLECTION OF BLOOD**
**Finger puncture**

MATERIALS:

Cotton balls
70% alcohol
Sterile blood lancet

PROCEDURE:

1. With cotton moistened with 70% alcohol, cleanse pad of finger.
2. With a piece of dry cotton, thoroughly dry pad of finger.
3. Pick up a sterile blood lancet and remove wrapper.
4. With right hand, firmly grasp sterile lancet.
5. With left hand, firmly grasp patient's middle finger.
6. With a quick drop and a quick rise of lancet, make *deep* stab on pad of finger.
7. Take a piece of dry cotton and wipe away first drop.
8. Form a large rounded drop of blood at site of puncture.
9. Perform tests desired.
10. Place a piece of cotton on puncture until bleeding stops.

**Venipuncture**

MATERIALS:

Cotton balls
70% alcohol
Tourniquet
Needle (20 gauge)
Vacutainer tube and holder

PROCEDURE:

1. Assemble Vacutainer shell and needle. (The diameter of a needle is given by its gauge number. The smaller the number, the greater the diameter.)
2. Apply tourniquet above bend in elbow.
3. Select vein.
4. Moisten a piece of cotton with 70% alcohol and thoroughly rub cotton on vein you have selected.
5. Select a proposed point of entry into vein. Now place left thumb about

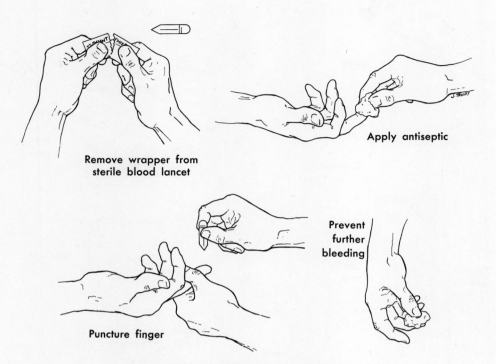

Remove wrapper from
sterile blood lancet

Apply antiseptic

Puncture finger

Prevent
further
bleeding

**Fig. 2-1.** Finger puncture technique.

2.5 cm (1 in) below this proposed point of entry. Press down firmly with thumb and pull skin toward yourself.
6. Point needle in exactly the same direction as vein is running.
7. Hold Vacutainer at a 15° angle and needle bevel up.
8. Push needle firmly and deliberately into vein.
9. Withdraw blood.
10. Release tourniquet.
11. Pick up a piece of cotton and gently hold it on puncture.
12. Withdraw needle.
13. When needle is out of arm, press cotton on puncture.

## ESTIMATION OF HEMOGLOBIN

Hemoglobin is a conjugated protein present in the red blood cells. It is responsible for the red color of blood. The prosthetic (nonprotein) compound combined with protein (globin) to form hemoglobin is called *heme.* Heme is an organic compound containing iron in chemical combination (iron porphyrin). This iron has a valence of +2 (ferrous iron).

It is the function of hemoglobin to combine loosely with oxygen in the lungs and to take it to the tissues, where a part of this oxygen is released. Hemoglobin combined with oxygen is called *oxyhemoglobin.* Oxyhemoglobin shows three absorption bands when scanned in a spectrophotometer (absorption at a wavelength of 578, 542, and 415 nm).

Methods for the determination of hemoglobin concentration of whole blood might be divided into two groups: primary and secondary methods. The primary methods are, for all practical purposes, too tedious and time consuming to

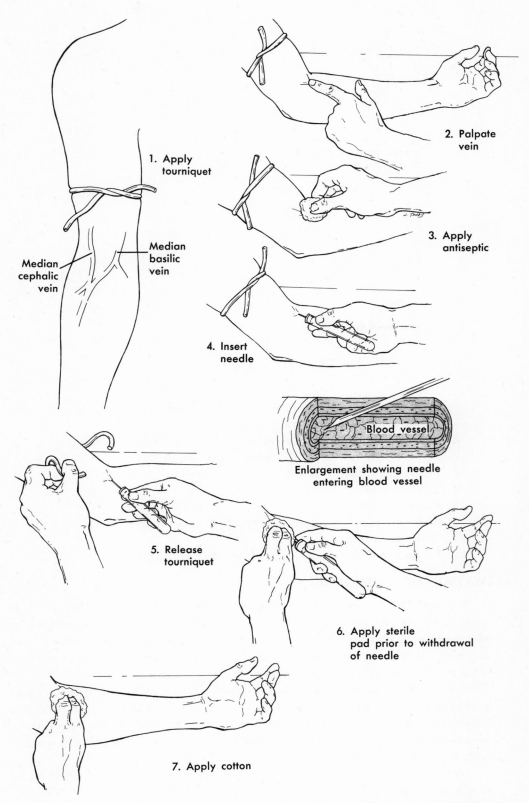

1. Apply
   tourniquet

Median
cephalic
vein

Median
basilic
vein

2. Palpate
   vein

3. Apply
   antiseptic

4. Insert
   needle

Blood vessel

Enlargement showing needle
entering blood vessel

5. Release
   tourniquet

6. Apply sterile
   pad prior to withdrawal
   of needle

7. Apply cotton

**Fig. 2-2.** Venipuncture technique.

be used as a routine method for hemoglobin analysis, but they have their value in that they can be used for the standardization of routine procedures (secondary methods). The properties of hemoglobin that serve in primary methods are essentially two: (1) the oxygen-combining property of hemoglobin and (2) the iron content of the hemoglobin molecule. Most of the secondary methods are based on spectral characteristics of hemoglobin or its derivatives.

Each gram of oxyhemoglobin is capable of combining with 1.34 volumes percent (vol%) of oxygen. Therefore if the oxygen capacity of blood is divided by 1.34, the quotient gives the number of grams of hemoglobin per 100 ml of blood. In fully oxygenated blood from a normal person there will be about 20.9 vol% of molecular oxygen. Therefore an average value of 15.6 of hemoglobin is present.

Each 100 g hemoglobin contains 335 mg iron. Therefore if the iron contained in 100 ml of blood is determined, and this value is divided by 3.35, the quotient equals the grams of hemoglobin per 100 ml of blood.

The blood oxygen capacity measures functional hemoglobin only and is inaccurate in that 2% to 12% of adult hemoglobin may be of an inactive form (unable to take up oxygen), which cannot be regenerated, and therefore it would not be measured by this method.

Total-blood-iron measurement for all practical purposes may be regarded as being bound to hemoglobin, the serum iron level being relatively small. Total-blood-iron analysis is considered the best method for the primary standardization of routine hemoglobin analysis.

## Cyanmethemoglobin method

PRINCIPLE: In the cyanmethemoglobin technique the blood specimen is diluted with Drabkin's reagent. The potassium ferricyanide converts hemoglobin iron from the ferrous state to the ferric state to form methemoglobin, which then combines with potassium cyanide to produce the stable pigment cyanmethemoglobin. The absorbance of the cyanmethemoglobin is then read at 540 nm.

MATERIALS:

1. Drabkin's reagent:
   1.0 g sodium bicarbonate
   0.05 g potassium cyanide
   0.20 g potassium ferricyanide
   Distilled water to 1 liter
   (This solution should be kept in brown bottle not longer than 1 month. The solution is clear and pale yellow. Discard if it appears turbid.)
2. 5 ml transfer pipette
   $20\lambda$ (0.02 ml) pipette
   Cuvettes
   Spectrophotometer

PROCEDURE:

1. Measure 5.0 ml Drabkin's reagent into cuvette.
2. Draw blood into a hemoglobin pipette until it is slightly above the 0.02 ml

mark. Wipe excess from outside of pipette and adjust exactly to 0.02 ml mark by touching tip of pipette to finger.

3. Blow blood into diluent and rinse pipette at least three times with diluent. Cover cuvette with parafilm and mix contents by inverting several times.
4. Let stand 5 min.
5. Adjust spectrophotometer to zero absorbance with cuvette filled with Drabkin's reagent at a wavelength of 540 nm.
6. Place cuvette containing blood sample in spectrophotometer. Read and record the reading.

CALCULATIONS: Transfer this reading to the standard curve and obtain the hemoglobin concentration in grams per deciliter of blood.

NORMAL VALUES:

Male:   15 to 19 g/dl (at 4400 ft)
        14 to 18 g/dl (at sea level)
Female: 13 to 17 g/dl (at 4400 ft)
        12 to 16 g/dl (at sea level)

## HEMATOCRIT

PRINCIPLE: The hematocrit is a test to determine the ratio of cells to fluid in blood. This test is generally considered more accurate than the red cell count.

MATERIALS: Capillary tubes (1 mm bore and approximately 75 mm in length): a blue-tipped tube does not contain any anticoagulant and is used when whole blood has already been treated with an anticoagulant. A red-tipped tube contains heparin and is used with capillary blood.

PROCEDURE:

1. Fill a capillary tube 2/3 to 3/4 full of blood. If using capillary blood, tilt tube back and forth to allow heparin to mix with blood and thus prevent coagulation.
2. Seal end of capillary tube with clay.
3. Centrifuge tube in a microhematocrit centrifuge at 12,000 rpm for 5 min.

CALCULATIONS: The volume of packed cells is expressed as a percentage of the total length of the column of blood. A special hematocrit reader is available for this measurement.

NORMAL VALUES:

Male:   45 to 51 (at 4400 ft)
        40 to 47 (at sea level)
Female: 40 to 49 (at 4400 ft)
        37 to 47 (at sea level)

## WHITE BLOOD CELL COUNT

PRINCIPLE: The diluting fluid hemolyses all nonnucleated red cells but does not alter leukocytes, thus facilitating enumeration of the white blood cells.

MATERIALS:

3% glacial acetic acid
White blood cell pipette
Hemacytometer counting chamber

PROCEDURE:

1. Draw blood slightly above 0.5 mark of white cell pipette. Wipe off outside of pipette and adjust blood exactly to 0.5 mark by touching pipette tip to finger.
2. Draw 3% acetic acid diluent to 11 mark.
3. Shake pipette (3 min by hand).
4. Expel and discard first 4 drops from pipette.
5. Place clean coverslip on counting chamber. Allow counting chamber area under coverslip to be completely filled with mixture.
6. Under low power, count number of leukocytes in each of the four large corner squares.

CALCULATIONS:

Dilution 1:20
Volume counts 4 per 10 cu mm
Number of cells counted $\times$ 10/4 $\times$ 20 = number of cells per cubic millimeter

NORMAL VALUES: 5000 to 10,000 per cu mm. Values above 11,000 are usually considered as representing leukocytosis, whereas those below 4000 indicate leukopenia.

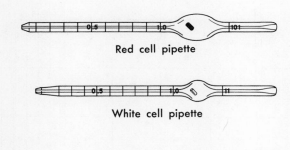

Red cell pipette

White cell pipette

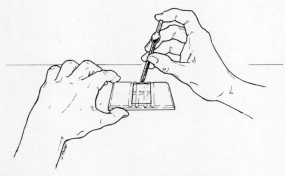

**Fig. 2-3.** Method for charging hemacytometer counting chamber.

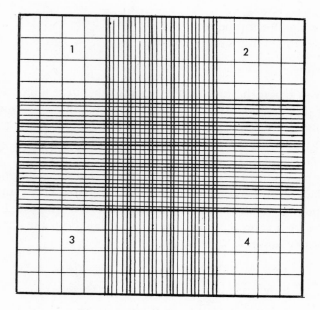

**Fig. 2-4.** The hemacytometer.

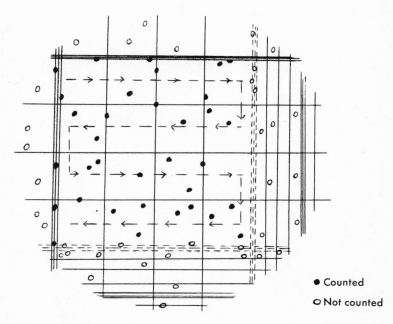

● Counted

○ Not counted

**Fig. 2-5.** Diagram of white cell count. A white cell is counted only once by counting those within the medium-sized square and those touching any line at the left and top, but not counting those at any line at the right and bottom of the medium-sized square. All cells touching the triple lines shown as broken lines will be excluded.

# DIFFERENTIAL LEUKOCYTE (WHITE BLOOD CELL) COUNT

PRINCIPLE: The purpose of the differential leukocyte count is to establish the relative frequency of each type of cell.

PROCEDURE:

1. After puncturing skin, remove and discard first drop of blood and touch one end of a slide to the small, newly formed drop. Place end of a second slide over drop of blood and smear across first slide.
2. Permit smear to air dry and flood it with Wright's stain for 1 min. Then add enough buffer to completely cover slide; let stand for 2 min while mixing stain, and buffer by blowing gently. Wash with distilled water until stain is removed. Blot dry.
3. Inspect smear under low power. Observe distribution of leukocytes and choose that portion of smear, usually near thin end, where there is no overlapping of erythrocytes. Shift to oil immersion objective.
4. Move slide from extreme upper edge of smear to extreme lower edge, counting and classifying each leukocyte in the successive fields. Shift over one field and proceed to upper edge, still classifying each leukocyte. Continue in this fashion until required number of cells is counted.
5. Always note and report morphology of erythrocytes and morphology and number of platelets. When platelet count is normal, an average of three to five platelets is seen per oil immersion field.

**Fig. 2-6.** Procedure for differential leukocyte counts of blood smears.

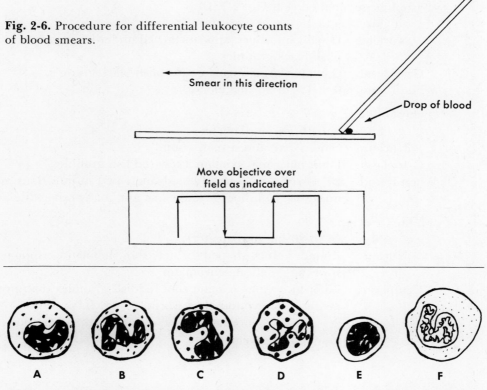

Smear in this direction

Drop of blood

Move objective over field as indicated

**Fig. 2-7. A,** Neutrophilic band cell. **B,** Neutrophilic segmented cell. **C,** Eosinophilic segmented cell. **D,** Basophilic segmented cell. **E,** Lymphocyte. **F,** Monocyte.

11

## White cells found in a normal differential white cell count

Neutrophilic band cell (Fig. 2-7, *A*)
Size: 9 to 15 μm in diameter
Nucleus: Shaped like a band
Cytoplasm: Contains small pink granules
When found: 2% to 6% in normal blood; increased in appendicitis, pneumonia, and many other diseases

Neutrophilic segmented cell (Fig. 2-7, *B*)
Size: 9 to 15 μm in diameter
Nucleus: Broken up into segments, connected by a thin strand of chromatin
Cytoplasm: Contains small pink granules
When found: 55% to 75% in normal blood; increased in appendicitis, pneumonia, and many other diseases

Eosinophilic segmented cell (Fig. 2-7, *C*)
Size: 9 to 15 μm in diameter
Nucleus: Usually has two lobes or segments
Cytoplasm: Contains large red granules
When found: 1% to 3% in normal blood; increased in asthma, hay fever, and parasitic infestations

Basophilic segmented cell (Fig. 2-7, *D*)
Size: 9 to 15 μm in diameter
Nucleus: Usually indistinct; appears buried under large purple or purplish black granules
Cytoplasm: Contains large purple or purplish black granules
When found: 0 to 1% in normal blood

Lymphocyte (Fig. 2-7, *E*)
Size: 8 to 16 μm in diameter
Nucleus: Closely knit and usually round
Cytoplasm: Light blue; may contain a few reddish granules
When found: 20% to 35% in normal blood; increased in infectious mononucleosis, lymphocytic leukemia, and many other diseases

Monocyte (Fig. 2-7, *F*)
Size: 14 to 20 μm in diameter
Nucleus: Round, kidney-shaped, or may show lobulation; spongy and sprawling, delicate chromatin
Cytoplasm: Light gray; may contain tiny reddish granules that give appearance of ground glass; vacuoles may be present
When found: 2% to 5% in normal blood; increased in tuberculosis and monocytic leukemia

**Table 1.** Increased cell percentage found in the more common diseases

| Lymphocytes | Monocytes | Eosinophilic cells | Neutrophilic cells | Basophilic cells |
|---|---|---|---|---|
| Mumps | Typhus | Asthma | Appendicitis | Polycythemia |
| Pertussis | Rocky | Hay fever | Pneumonia | vera |
| Whooping | Mountain | Scarlet fever | Tonsillitis | Ulcerative |
| cough | spotted | Parasitic | Acute hemor- | colitis |
| Thyrotoxico- | fever | infestations | rhage | Smallpox |
| sis | Tuberculosis | Chronic | Granulocytic | Nephrosis |
| Infectious | Hodgkin's | granulocytic | leukemia | Myxedema |
| mononucle- | disease | leukemia | | Chronic |
| osis | Monocytic | Pernicious | | granulocytic |
| Lymphocytic | leukemia | anemia | | leukemia |
| leukemia | | | | |

*See worksheets, pp. 77-81.*

# 3 Introduction to immunohematology

SANDRA V. CULLIMORE, M.T. (ASCP)SBB

Blood is a complex tissue composed of formed elements—red cells, white cells, and platelets—suspended in the liquid, plasma. The study of blood is termed hematology.

The healing powers of blood have intrigued man since the beginning of time. Egyptian history records the use of blood baths for treating the ill. And in the Roman Empire it was the practice of spectators to drink the blood of the dying gladiators in an attempt to obtain some of their strength. However, blood transfusion as we know it was not performed until the seventeenth century.

With the discovery of the circulatory system, some of the mysterious properties of blood were understood, and intravenous (within the vein) blood transfusion became possible.

In 1667 a French physician named Denys attempted a direct transfusion from the carotid artery of a lamb into the cubital vein of a human. This seemed successful until the experiment was repeated—with disastrous results. His description of the patient experiencing "fever, chill and voiding blackish colored urine" is probably the first recorded hemolytic transfusion reaction. In this type of blood reaction the injected red blood cells dissolve in the patient's bloodstream and are passed as hemoglobin products in the urine. The destruction of these cells causes the sudden, extreme symptoms and can cause irreversible damage to the kidneys, resulting in prolonged suffering and even death.

With the realization of the obvious incompatibility of blood from one species to another, this practice of animal to human transfusion was prohibited. Several years later, in 1818, an English obstetrician successfully transfused small amounts of human blood into a patient suffering from acute blood loss. The results were remarkable. However, there followed some severe reactions of human to human blood, and it became evident there were some intraspecies differences to be resolved.

Another major difficulty encountered was that of coagulation or normal blood clotting. To transfuse blood it would be necessary to maintain it in the liquid state. Numerous devices were invented to attempt to remove fibrin strands as they formed in the blood. Other experiments involved adding chemicals that would prevent coagulation.

In 1914 a suitable chemical was found that could be added to the blood, would prevent clotting, and yet would not harm the patient. This solution is ACD (acid-citrate-dextrose), which acts not only as an anticoagulant but also has

**14**

nutrient and preservative properties for the red cells. A phosphate-buffered modification of the original formula is now available as CPD. This solution in normal amounts is harmless to the recipient and is metabolized by the body following the transfusion.

## HUMAN BLOOD GROUPS

Dr. Karl Landsteiner has been called the "father of immunohematology" for his discovery of the ABO blood groups. His experiments involving samples of serum and red cells led to the basic theory of antigen (on the cell) and antibody (in the serum) reactions in immunohematology (the study of these antigen-antibody reactions in the blood).

In discussing antigen we must first imagine antibody as a portion of the globulins or proteins in serum or plasma capable of combining in some observable way with its specific antigen (substance that generated the production of the immune bodies or antibodies).

In recognition of a foreign invading material (antigen), the individual creates antibody directed against the recognized non-self antigen. The acceptance by our immune system of our own antigens and rejection of foreign antigen led Dr. Landsteiner to his statement, which is often referred to as Landsteiner's rule: "If the antigen is present in the individual's genetic structure, antibody [against that particular antigen] will be absent from his serum" (Fig. 3-1).

Or stating this phenomenon another way, we might say that if antibody is present in the serum of an individual, its causative antigen will not be part of his own genetic structure (Fig. 3-2).

As a result of Dr. Landsteiner's discoveries and through the production of

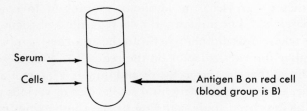

**Fig. 3-1.** Serum will not contain anti-B (B antigen is "self") because antigen B is present in patient's genetic structure. Patient is classified as blood group B.

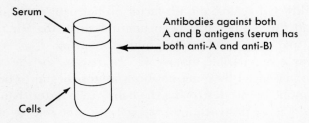

**Fig. 3-2.** Patient's serum is tested and found to contain antibodies against both A and B antigens (serum has both anti-A and anti-B). Therefore his red cells must possess neither A nor B antigens. Patient is classified as blood group O.

**15**

natural antibodies to A or B antigens by humans, we can classify blood samples into four major blood groups:

| Group | Antigens (on cells) | Antibodies (in serum) |
|-------|---------------------|------------------------|
| A | A | Anti-B |
| B | B | Anti-A |
| AB | A and B | Neither anti-A nor anti-B |
| O | Neither | Anti-A and anti-B |

These natural antibodies to A or B (depending on which is recognized as foreign) are apparently the result of our exposure during the first few months after birth to animal and plant products having A or B antigens. We accept the self antigens and create antibodies against those we recognize as different or foreign.

## THE Rh SYSTEM

The discovery of the ABO blood group system opened the way for recognizing the myriad factors that may be present on red blood cells as inherited characteristics. Many research scientists in the field of immunohematology have made remarkable discoveries and contributed much to our present knowledge of the blood groups.

The most significant discovery since ABO is that of the Rh factor. This characteristic is named for the *rhesus* monkey whose red cells served as the antigen in animal immunization studies performed in about 1940.

The animal antibody was called anti-rhesus (or anti-Rh), and it was observed that serum from some mothers whose infants suffered from newborn jaundice contained antibody that seemed to be similar if not identical to the anti-Rh animal antibody.

As studies progressed, the antibody was found to react with a majority (approximately 85%) of human red cells regardless of their A or B characteristics. Those whose cells did not react with the anti-rhesus antibody were classified as Rh negative (no rhesus factor on the red cells). With increased knowledge it has been shown that the rhesus factor and human Rh factor are not identical but very similar. Chemical and structural similarities of various antigens have been the basis for improved understanding of the complexities of immunohematology.

In some but not all of the Rh-negative mothers tested, an anti-Rh antibody was detected. In keeping with Landsteiner's rule, her own red cells did not contain the antigen against which she had developed serum antibody. Her antibody was directed against the Rh factor on her baby's cells (inherited from the father), and the mother had been immunized to the Rh factor through her pregnancy and delivery of an Rh-positive offspring.

This was a remarkable discovery. The reason for the severe anemia and jaundice experienced by some newborn infants began to be understood. The maternal antibody was destroying the baby's cells faster than he could produce more. This massive destruction of red cells with the release of their hemoglobin was more than the child's liver could handle, and allowing the bilirubin (product of hemoglobin destruction) to be reabsorbed was causing the jaundiced appearance of the newborn.

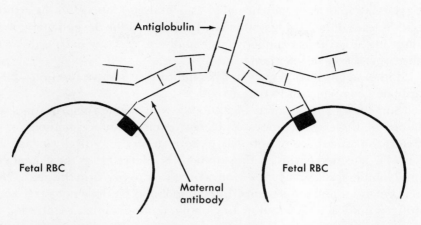

**Fig. 3-3.** Antihuman globulin detects maternal serum globulin (anti-Rh), which is itself adhering to the Rh antigen site on the infant's red cells.

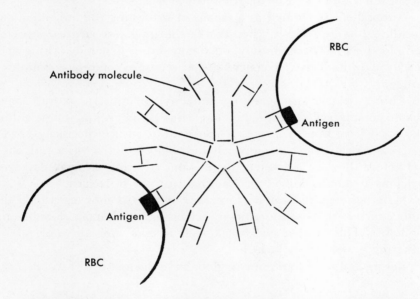

**Fig. 3-4.** Agglutination of red cells (antigen) by antibody molecule.

The Coombs test became a valuable aid in diagnosing whether an infant was likely to develop this newborn jaundice. The maternal anti-Rh antibody could be found adhering to the infant's Rh-positive red cells when the test was done using the anti-human globulin reagent (Fig. 3-3).

## ANTIGEN-ANTIBODY REACTIONS

Antigens such as the A and B factors are sometimes called *agglutinogens* and their antibodies, anti-A and anti-B, are called *agglutinins*. These names are derived from the characteristic reaction observed when they combine, namely agglutination or a clumping together of the red cells in irregular aggregates as a result of antibody adhering to antigen sites on two or more cells that are in close proximity (Fig. 3-4).

As we observe other reactions in immunohematology, they will be either

**17**

agglutination or they may be noted as hemolysis (damage to the cell membrane with release of its hemoglobin). The hemolysis is the development of a pink-red tinge in the serum as antibody (an hemolysin) reacts with its cellular antigen in the presence of serum complement.

Either agglutination or hemolysis indicates a positive reaction—that antigen-antibody combination has occurred.

Sometimes the reaction of antibody with antigen will be undetectable by either of these observations and may require indirect methods of testing to detect the adherence of antibody to antigen on the red cell surface.

The detection of this coating antibody is referred to as the Coombs test or the antiglobulin test. A reagent serum is necessary to perform this test. This Coombs reagent is an antibody against human globulin. It does not react with red cell antigen but will attach to human globulin (antibody) that is adhering to red cell antigen.

The appearance of agglutination at completion of this test indicates a positive Coombs test and could be diagrammed as in Fig. 3-5.

Antibodies are formed as a means of protecting the individual against the invading, foreign antigen, whether it be the antigen of viruses, of bacteria, or of red blood cells. The immunity, once initiated, is generally lasting and may be reactivated with increased activity (hyperimmunity) on repeat stimulus with that antigen.

Antiserum (serum containing antibody) or antisera (plural) may be purchased commercially and used to determine blood groups. These antibodies are extracted from human serum, are purified (to insure specificity), and are evaluated to measure the concentration and ability to detect weak antigens (sensitivity) before they are marketed. Regulations covering the manufacture of these reagents are controlled by the National Institute of Health.

Materials required for performance of the Coombs test would include an animal serum with specific antibody activity against human globulin (antihuman globulin). This reagent will react wtih human globulin molecules that are adhering to red cell surfaces.

Before adding the antihuman globulin to the mixture of serum and cells, the

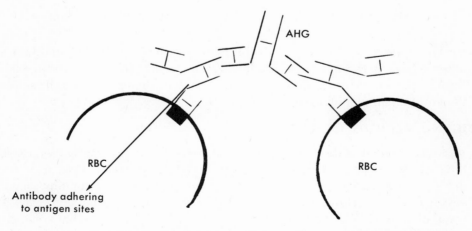

**Fig. 3-5.** The antiglobulin (Coombs) test. AHG (antihuman globulin) reacts with human globulin (antibody), which is attached to its antigen site on the red cell.

18

cells must be washed with normal saline. This washing will remove excess globulin, which, if left with the cells, would neutralize the antihuman globulin before it can detect the cell-bound globulin (antibody). A false-negative Coombs test would result, and we would not know whether the cells were coated with antibody (globulin).

## USES OF ANTIGEN-ANTIBODY REACTIONS

The field of immunohematology is in a state of constant change as new discoveries and improved testing techniques become available. The determination of ABO group, Rh type, and the performance of the antiglobulin (Coombs) test are some of the most basic yet most important tests one can perform.

Special typing in medicolegal cases, solving unusual antibody problems in transfusion candidates, or identifying the antibody affecting the cells of a newborn infant are interesting and rewarding experiences for the medical technologist. A mistake could jeopardize the patient's life. The need for careful application of the principles of immunohematology confers a tremendous responsibility on the blood-bank technologist.

## CELL GROUPING
### Forward grouping

PRINCIPLE: The ABO blood groups are determined by testing the red cells against known anti-A, anti-B, and anti-A, B antisera. The $Rh_0(D)$ typing is determined by testing the red cells against known anti-$Rh_0(D)$ antisera.

PROCEDURE:

1. Divide three glass slides in half using a wax pencil.
2. Label the divisions anti-A, anti-B, anti-A,B, anti-D, and control.
3. Place one drop of anti-A, anti-B, and anti-A,B into respective squares.
4. With new applicator stick, add small amount of blood to each square.
5. With new applicator stick, mix cells and antisera.
6. Tilt slide and observe for agglutination. (Do *not* warm.)
7. Onto third slide place one drop anti-D and one drop 22% bovine albumin.
8. With new applicator stick, add small amount of blood to each square.
9. With new applicator stick, mix cells and antisera.
10. Place glass slide on warm viewing box glass and tilt slide back and forth for 2 min.
11. Examine for agglutination.

INTERPRETATION:

| Anti-A | Anti-B | Anti-A, B | Blood group |
|--------|--------|-----------|-------------|
| + | − | + | A |
| − | + | + | B |
| + | + | + | AB |
| − | − | − | O |

| Anti-D | Control | $Rh_0(D)$ type |
|--------|---------|----------------|
| + | − | Positive |
| − | − | Negative |

## Reverse grouping

PRINCIPLE: Reverse grouping is used as a check on the accuracy of ABO grouping performed on the red cells. The test is performed by examining the serum of the patient or donor against reagent red blood cells. Consisting of known $A_1$ Rh-negative and B Rh-negative red cells, they will reveal the presence or absence of anti-A or anti-B isoagglutinins. Whenever A or B blood group antigen is absent from the red cells, the corresponding isoagglutinin is normally present in the serum.

PROCEDURE:

1. Prepare a set of two tubes for each unknown serum to be tested (label $A_1$, B). To each of the two tubes add 2 drops of patient's serum.
2. To tubes labeled $A_1$, add 1 drop of $A_1$ cells, and to tubes labeled B, add 1 drop of B cells.
3. Centrifuge all tubes at 3400 rpm for 15 seconds, examine for agglutination, and record results.

INTERPRETATION:

| $A_1$ cells | B cells | Blood group |
|-------------|---------|-------------|
| − | + | A |
| + | − | B |
| − | − | AB |
| + | + | O |

## ANTIGLOBULIN (COOMBS) TEST

PRINCIPLE: The antiglobulin test has evolved as the principal serologic procedure for the detection and the identification of in vivo and in vitro antigen-antibody complexes that do not agglutinate in saline.

The antibody test is dependent on the attachment of specific serum globulins onto specific antigen sites that are present on red blood cells after a suitable period of incubation. When the red cells are washed free of the surrounding serum proteins and antihuman globulin serum is added, the sensitized red cells are aggregated.

The antihuman globulin serum is produced by injecting rabbits with human serum. Coombs and co-workers showed that the rabbit antibody produced in response to the human gamma globulin would react with any incomplete antibody attached to a cell surface. These intercellular bridges, made of rabbit antibody to gamma globulin, link together red cells coated with human incomplete isoantibodies into large visible aggregates.

The direct antiglobulin test, which is used to detect the in vivo sensitization of erythrocytes, is a useful aid in establishing the diagnosis of hemolytic disease of the newborn, hemolytic anemia due to the autoimmune diseases, and hemolytic anemia induced by drug and antibiotic therapy.

The indirect antiglobulin test is used for detection and identification of irregular or immune antibodies of the IgG classification.

### Direct antiglobulin test

PROCEDURE:

1. Place 2 drops of red blood cells in a 10 × 75 mm test tube. Wash cells four times with physiologic saline.
2. Add 2 drops of antiglobulin serum to tube. Mix thoroughly.
3. Centrifuge.
4. Gently resuspend cell button and observe macroscopically for agglutination.

### Indirect antiglobulin test

PROCEDURE:

1. Place 2 drops of serum to be tested in each of two 10 × 75 mm test tubes. Label tubes I and II.
2. Add 1 drop of screening cells I and II to respective tubes.
3. Centrifuge immediately.
4. Resuspend red cell button and observe macroscopically for agglutination or hemolysis.
5. Add 2 drops albumin to tubes.
6. Incubate tubes in a 37°C water bath for 30 min.
7. Centrifuge tubes and observe for agglutination.
8. Wash red cells thoroughly with saline four times. Decant last washing so that cell button appears to be dry.
9. Add 2 drops of antihuman globulin serum. Mix thoroughly.
10. Centrifuge immediately and observe for agglutination.

INTERPRETATION: Agglutination of the red cells in the direct antiglobulin test indicates that they have been coated with antibody *in vivo*. Agglutination of the red cells in the indirect antiglobulin test indicates that the serum being tested contains an antibody.


*See worksheets, pp. 83-90.*

# 4 Coagulation

## CAPILLARY RESISTANCE TEST

PRINCIPLE: The capillary resistance test is often referred to as the capillary fragility test, the tourniquet test, or the Rumpel-Leede test.

The capillary resistance test measures the ability of the capillaries to resist pressure. In health the capillaries in the arm will resist a pressure of 100 mm Hg. In thrombocytopenic purpura, however, the capillaries in the arm will break or rupture after a pressure of 100 mm Hg. Tiny spots will then appear. These spots are hemorrhages or petechiae.

Conditions accompanied by a positive capillary resistance test include

1. Thrombocytopenic purpura
2. Vitamin K deficiency
3. Scurvy
4. Chronic nephritis
5. Measles
6. Influenza
7. Scarlet fever

PROCEDURE:

1. Take patient's blood pressure.
2. Inflate pressure cuff to halfway between diastolic and systolic pressure and maintain for 5 min.
3. Release pressure and allow 10 min to elapse.
4. Observe and record petechiae in an area on forearm about size of a quarter.

NORMAL: Less than 10 petechiae.

## BLEEDING TIME (DUKE'S METHOD)

PRINCIPLE: Conditions accompanied by an abnormal bleeding time include

1. Thrombocytopenic purpura
2. Hemorrhagic disease of the newborn
3. Scurvy
4. Allergy
5. Aplastic anemia
6. Pernicious anemia
7. Acute leukemia
8. Hodgkin's disease
9. Multiple myeloma
10. Infectious mononucleosis

PROCEDURE:

1. Use a sharp lancet to puncture earlobe or finger to depth of 3 mm. Start stopwatch.

2. At half-minute intervals, gently apply edge of small disk of filter paper to drop of blood—do not touch skin. Use a fresh edge of filter paper disk for each half-minute blotting.
3. Time in minutes equals number of blots divided by 2.

NORMAL: 1 to 3 min.

*See worksheet, p. 91.*

# 5 Clinical cytogenetics

**CELL DIVISION**
**Mitosis**

Mitosis is the mechanism by which somatic cells multiply. In mitosis each dividing cell produces two daughter cells, each of which has the exact chromosome complement as the parent cell.

Women have two X chromosomes. One is inherited from their mother and one from their father. Men have one X and one Y chromosome. The Y chromosome is inherited from their father and the X from their mother. Women have 23 pairs of homologous chromosomes, whereas men have only 22 pairs because their sex chromosomes are not alike. Apparently the combined action of some genes in both X chromosomes is required to produce a fertile woman, and the action of some genes in the Y chromosomes is required to produce a fertile man.

**Meiosis**

Meiosis is the mechanism by which gametes (ova and sperm) with a haploid complement of chromosomes are produced from their diploid parent cells. The daughter cells of a mitotic division are diploid (2N). Those of a meiotic division are haploid (N).

**Abnormalities of chromosomes**

**Crossing-over.** Crossing-over is an exchange of genetic material between homologous chromosomes during prophase of the first meiotic division.

**Nondisjunction.** Nondisjunction is the failure of a pair of homologous chromosomes to separate and migrate to different cells during anaphase of cell division. Meiotic disjunction occurs twice (meiosis I or meiosis II), so there is twice as much opportunity for nondisjunction or premature disjunction as there is during mitotic division.

Nondisjunction during meiosis I produces only abnormal gametes; nondisjunction during meiosis II yields equal numbers of both normal and abnormal gametes. Nondisjunction that affects either meiosis I or meiosis II is called primary nondisjunction. When nondisjunction occurs in an individual who already has a chromosomal abnormality as a result of a previous nondisjunction, it is termed secondary nondisjunction.

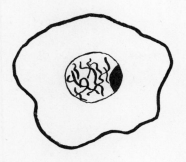

**Fig. 5-1.** The sex chromatin body or Barr body.

## SEX CHROMATIN TESTS

There are two types of sex chromatin tests: epithelial chromatin "Barr body" tests and neutrophil "drumstick" (appendages seen on the segmented nucleus of the neutrophil) tests.

Examination of epithelial cell nuclei for the characteristic sex chromatin (Barr) body is known as the sex chromatin test or Barr test. In smears from normal women and girls the Barr body is seen in 40% to 60% of nuclei.

The sex chromatin body originates from one whole inactivated X chromosome. The experimental evidence for this view was presented by Dr. M. F. Lyon, and the concept is therefore known as the Lyon hypothesis. According to the Lyon hypothesis, all X chromosomes in excess of one are inactivated (heterochromatinized) and form nuclear chromatin masses. The number of Barr bodies in any cell is therefore $n-1$, where $n$ is the number of X chromosomes present. It is important to remember that Barr tests do not determine genetic sex. Genetic sex depends on the presence or absence of a Y chromosome and not on the number of X chromosomes present. The proper way to report these tests is chromatin negative or chromatin positive. Variations in number of Barr bodies in each nucleus, the percentage of chromatin-positive cells, and the size of the Barr body should also be reported.

### Buccal smear preparation

PROCEDURE:

1. Scrape buccal mucosa with spatula, discard, scrape again, and spread on one slide. Cover with second slide and press firmly together.
2. Slide the slides apart and place immediately into stain.
3. Stain with alcoholic Giemsa for 2 min.
4. Buffer for 1 min with 40 ml distilled water buffered to pH 6.0 to 6.5 with 5 ml dibasic sodium phosphate.
5. Clear in acetone for 10 sec.
6. Clear in acetone:xylene (1:1) solution for 10 sec.
7. Clear in xylene for 1 min.
8. Carefully blot dry.

NOTE: Always do both right and left sides of cheek. Always run a known-positive female control with sample to be analyzed to assure validity of test.

*See worksheet, p. 93.*

# 6 Urinalysis

From earliest times, abnormalities of urine have been associated with disease. It was noted that insects were attracted to certain urines, which usually suggested sugar was present in that urine.

In the early seventeenth century there were practitioners of uromancy called *pisse-prophets*. They tried to diagnose diseases by simply looking at the patient's urine.

In 1827 at Guy's Hospital in London, Richard Bright made urine testing a part of regular medical examinations, and in the early 1900s Thomas Addis further advanced the art by advocating the study of urine sediment. An important part of this workup is the urinalysis—and it is a relatively easy sample to obtain. Yet in most laboratories it is the urinalysis department that is put in the far corner of the furnace room, and to work there is considered a form of punishment.

Urinalysis can be fascinating as well as of great diagnostic value. There are three major reasons for performing urinalysis:
1. Screen: screening groups of people for unsuspected disorders
2. Diagnose: relating urine abnormalities to other signs and symptoms for diagnosis
3. Monitor: monitoring the course of treatment of disease to identify effectiveness

## PHYSICAL ANALYSIS

The fresh, voided specimen is the best to examine. Since the nature of the sediment and chemical composition soon changes, the urine must be examined while fresh, preferably within 3 hours after it is voided. Note and record color, transparency, and specific gravity.

| Color | Usual cause |
|---|---|
| Straw to amber | Urochrome, a pigment found in normal urine |
| Colorless | Reduced concentration |
| Silvery sheen or milky | Pus, bacteria, or epithelial cells |
| Smoky brown | Blood |
| Black | Melanin |
| Port-wine | Porphyrins |
| Yellow foam | Bile or medications |
| Orange, green, blue, or red | Medications |

**Transparency.** The degree of transparency depends on the amount of suspended materials. Report as clear or cloudy.

After recording the transparency, centrifuge urine for 5 min at 1800 rpm before proceeding with specific gravity and chemical analysis.

**Specific gravity.** To make a specific gravity determination of urine, first clean surface of cover and prism of a refractometer (TS meter) with a damp cloth and then dry. Close cover. Apply a drop of urine at notched bottom of cover so that it flows over prism surface by capillary action. Point instrument toward light source at an angle that gives optimum contrast. Read directly on specific gravity scale and sharp dividing line between light and dark contrast.

Because of its dissolved substances, urine weighs more than water, the normal specific gravity being 1.008 to 1.030. Increased values are found in acute nephritis, fevers, and diabetes mellitus (because of dissolved sugar). Decreased values are found in chronic nephritis and diabetes insipidus (because of copious volume).

## CHEMICAL ANALYSIS
### Dipstick reading

Immerse all reagent areas of strip in urine and remove immediately. Tap edge of strip against side of urine container to remove excess urine. Compare test areas closely with corresponding color charts on bottle label at the times specified.

**pH reaction.** The pH of urine is a reflection of the ability of the kidney to maintain normal hydrogen ion concentration in plasma and extracellular fluid. In health, urine pH may range from pH 4.6 to pH 8.0. When protein intake is high, more phosphate and sulfates are produced. This results in more acid urine. On a predominantly vegetable diet, the urine may have a pH higher than 6.0. The urine becomes less acid following a meal as a result of secretion of acid into the stomach, the so-called alkaline tide. At night, during the mild respiratory acidosis of sleep, a more acid urine may be formed. The test area permits differentiation of pH values to half a unit within the range of 5.0 to 9.0.

**Ketone bodies.** In ketonuria the three ketone bodies present in urine are acetoacetic acid (20%), acetone (2%), and betahydroxybutyric acid (about 78%). Ketone bodies are the products of incomplete fat metabolism, and their presence indicates acidosis. Ketonuria is commonly seen in uncontrolled diabetes mellitus.

The test area detects 5 to 10 mg acetoacetic acid per 100 ml of urine. It is less sensitive to acetone and does not react with betahydroxybutyric acid.

Report as negative, 1+, 2+, 3+.

**Glucose.** Glucose occurs in the urine when the blood sugar is elevated and exceeds the renal threshold or when there is a lowered renal threshold.

The test area detects approximately 0.1% glucose. If positive on the dipstick, do the Clinitest method:

1. Place 5 drops urine in a test tube.
2. Add 10 drops distilled water.
3. Add 1 Clinitest tablet.
4. Report test as negative, trace, 1+, 2+, 3+, 4+.

**Occult blood.** Because of the diagnostic importance of small amounts of hematuria and because of the tendency of red blood cells to undergo lysis in urine, a screening test for hemoglobinuria is a useful adjunct to the microscopic examination of the sediment.

Report as negative, 1+, 2+, 3+.

**Bilirubin.** Free or unconjugated bilirubin is not able to pass through the glomerular barrier of the kidney. When free bilirubin is conjugated in the liver with glucuronic acid, it becomes water soluble and is able to pass through the glomerulus of the kidney. Conjugated bilirubin is normally excreted in the bile. In patients with obstructive jaundice, bilirubin is found in the urine; urine with yellow foam may accompany pale acholic stools.

The test area will not read positive below 0.2 mg/dl in urine.

Report as negative, 1+, 2+, 3+.

**Urobilinogen.** Conjugated bilirubin secreted by the liver into the bile is excreted through the bile ducts into the intestinal tract. In the intestinal tract the bilirubin is converted by bacterial action to a group of compounds known as urobilinogen. Approximately 40% to 50% of this urobilinogen can be reabsorbed into the portal circulation and reexcreted by the liver. Increased amounts in the urine are found in any condition that causes an increase in bilirubin production or any disease that prevents the liver from normally removing the reabsorbed urobilinogen from the portal circulation.

The test area will detect urobilinogen in concentrations of approximately 0.1 Ehrlich unit per 100 ml urine.

Report as negative, 1, 4, 8, 12 Ehrlich units per deciliter urine.

### Albumin (protein) determination

To about 2 ml urine supernatant, add approximately 8 drops of 20% sulfo-salicylic acid. Let stand 1 min. If albumin is present, a white cloud will form.

Report as negative, trace, 1+, 2+, 3+, 4+, depending on the amount of precipitate.

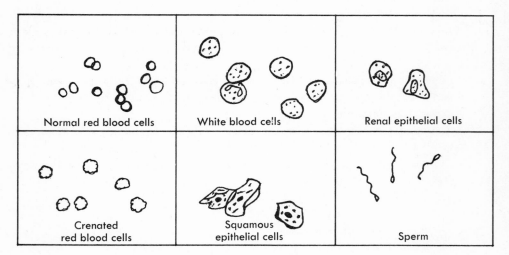

**Fig. 6-1.** Cells found in urine.

## MICROSCOPIC EXAMINATION

Loosen sediment by gently shaking or tapping bottom of tube. Place sediment on a glass slide. Examine under microscope, first under low power with reduced light, and list number and type of casts on average present. Next turn to high dry lens and examine urine.

Report number of WBCs and RBCs present per high power field. Report

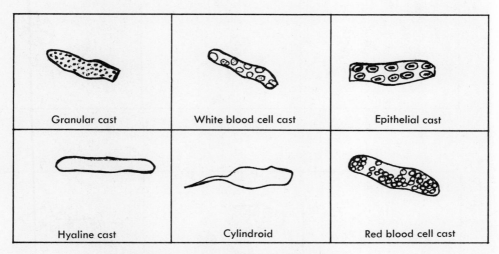

**Fig. 6-2.** Casts found in urinary sediment.

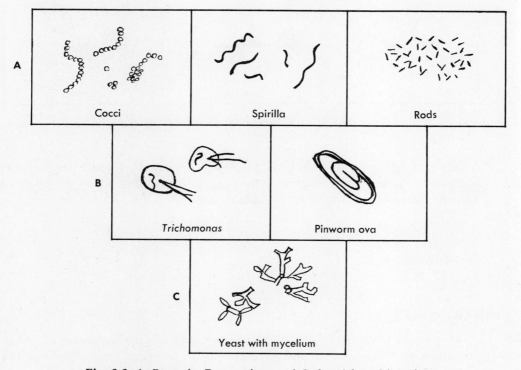

**Fig. 6-3. A,** Bacteria; **B,** parasites; and **C,** fungi found in urine.

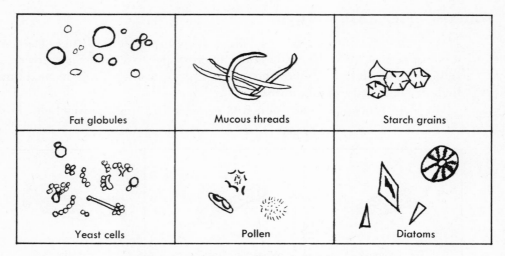

**Fig. 6-4.** Extraneous substances found in urine.

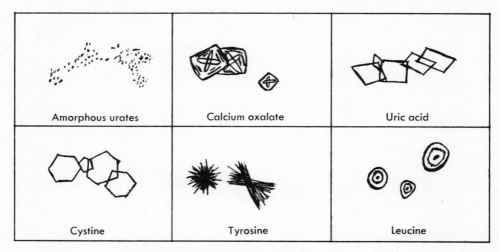

**Fig. 6-5.** Crystals found in acid urine.

number of epithelial cells as few, moderate, or many. Identify and report presence of renal epithelial cells if they are present. Also report presence of mucous threads, type of crystals, and bacteria.

*See worksheet, p. 95.*

## URINARY CALCULI

One of the major disorders of the urinary system is the formation of calculi (urolithiasis). Calculi are deposited chemicals in compact form. These stones may originate in the kidney and then pass into the ureter, or they may originate

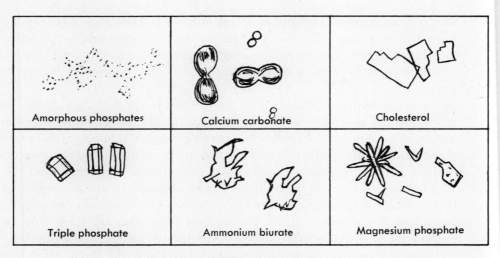

**Fig. 6-6.** Crystals found in alkaline urine.

in the bladder. Stones are composed of one or several chemical constituents: calcium, oxalate, phosphorus, magnesium, ammonium, cystine, and uric acid.

Calculi are classified as primary or secondary. The primary stones are those formed without apparent causal factors, such as infection, inflammation, or urinary obstruction and stasis. Secondary stones are those that follow evident inflammation or obstruction.

The cause of stone formation is unknown, but there are several factors that seem to contribute. The presence of two or more of these factors is usually associated with stone formation.

1. Metabolic disturbances
2. Urinary obstruction
3. Endocrinopathies
4. Infections
5. Mucosal metaplasia
6. Isohydruria (loss of the normal acid, alkaline tides, or a fixation of pH)
7. Extrinsic conditions (dehydration, dietary excess, drug excess, chemotherapy)

Although the presence of one of these factors usually will not cause stone formation, isohydruria is found most often in association with one or more of the other findings.

Urinary reaction (pH) is important in the maintenance of urinary salts in solution and largely determines the composition of the stones. Uric acid and cystine stones form in acid urine. Calcium oxalate stones form in a slightly acid to neutral pH; whereas phosphate stones occur in a neutral to slightly alkaline pH. Prolonged isohydruria favors the formation of pure calculi; calculi of mixed composition are found in patients showing a temporary and wide fluctuation of urinary pH.

Many calculi contain a clearly defined nucleus on which the chemicals precipitate. Solid material such as bacteria, tiny blood clots, necrotic or degenerated tissue, or other foreign bodies, may become encrusted with urinary salts. A

**31**

matrix composed of mucoproteins and mucopolysaccharides is reported to be present throughout the stone. This fibrous matrix surrounds the center of the calculus at a series of spaced intervals and is an essential factor in the initial phase of calculi formation and a determining factor in the position of crystal deposits.

Clinical manifestations vary with the size and location of the calculus. Small, smooth stones may be passed without any difficulty. Large stones may remain stationary within the renal pelvis for years without symptoms or with only intermittent lumbar discomfort. When a stone enters the ureter it may obstruct the outflow of urine, promote infection, and cause the pain of renal colic.

The size of a calculus ranges from very small gravel to a large staghorn stone that may fill the renal pelvis. Pure calculi, those containing only one compound, are found in approximately 30% to 40% of the calculi analyzed. Most calculi contain one or two principal constituents that are of interest to the clinician. The composition is somewhat dependent on the location of the stone. Adult bladder stones are composed chiefly of uric acid; whereas kidney stones are generally composed of calcium oxalate, triple phosphate (calcium, magnesium, ammonium phosphate), or apatite (calcium phosphate complexed with carbonate), or all three. Cystine stones are uncommon or of varying mixtures of cystine with phosphate and uric acids.

Stones have a number of distinguishing features according to their constituents. Uric acid stones are brown, fairly smooth, moderately hard, and show concentric laminations. Calcium oxalate stones are very hard and have a rough, spiny surface of dark brown color. Phosphate stones are soft, smooth, and white. Staghorn calculi are irregular and pronged in shape. They are usually associated with infection and are composed of phosphate, oxalate, and uric acid.

Various methods have been utilized in the analysis of calculi: x-ray diffraction, infrared spectrophotometry, chemical analysis, optical analysis, electron microscopy, electron diffraction, and thermoluminescence. At the present time the chemical method is still the method of choice in the clinical laboratory, since it is simple and accurate, requires no special equipment, and uses reagents that are readily available.

## Calculi analysis (Oxford Stone Analysis Kit)

PROCEDURE:

1. Into a 10 × 75 mm tube place a small (covering bottom of tube) amount of powdered stone.
2. Add 10 drops hydrochloric acid. Effervescence at this point indicates presence of carbonate ion.
3. Place 1 drop of this acid extract onto each of six spots in a glass spot-plate.
4. To one of the drops of acid extract, add 1 drop sodium cyanide. Mix and wait 5 min. Add 1 drop cystine reagent. A red color indicates presence of cystine. A yellow color indicates absence of cystine.
5. To another drop of acid extract, add 2 drops inorganic phosphate reagent. Mix and wait 5 min. A blue color indicates presence of inorganic phosphate. If no color change occurs, inorganic phosphate is absent.
6. To a third drop of acid, add 1 drop magnesium reagent and 5 drops

sodium hydroxide. Mix. A blue precipitate indicates presence of magnesium ion. A purple color with no precipitate indicates absence of magnesium ion.

7. Add 1 drop sodium hydroxide to another drop of acid extract. Then add 2 drops calcium reagent. Mix. A yellow color indicates presence of calcium ion. An orange color indicates absence of calcium ion.

8. To determine the presence of ammonium ion, add 1 drop sodium hydroxide and 1 drop ammonia reagent to a drop of acid extract. Mix. An orange color with brown precipitate indicates presence of ammonium ion. A yellow color indicates absence of ammonium ion.

9. To last drop of acid extract, add 1 drop sodium hydroxide and 1 drop uric acid reagent. Mix. A yellow-orange color indicates presence of urates or uric acid. No color change indicates absence of urates or uric acid.

10. To acid extract remaining in tube, add 2 drops oxalate reagent. Mix and wait 1 min. If bubbles do not develop immediately, observe carefully for 5 min. before recording reaction as negative. Slow, tiny bubbles indicate presence of oxalate.

*See worksheet, p. 97.*

# 7 Chemistry

**MATHEMATICS FOR MEDICAL TECHNOLOGISTS**
**Percentage solutions**

1. % w/v (w/v = grams of solute in 100 ml of solution)
2. % w/w (w/w = grams of solute in 100 g of solution)
3. % v/v (v/v = milliliters of solute in 100 ml of solution)

To prepare 100 ml of a 4% w/v solution of glucose:
1. Add 4 g glucose to a 100 ml volumetric flask.
2. Dissolve in distilled water.
3. Dilute to 100 ml.

What weight of fructose is needed to prepare 250 ml of an 8% w/v solution?

1. $\dfrac{8 \text{ g fructose}}{100 \text{ ml solution}}$

2. $\dfrac{8 \text{ g}}{100 \text{ ml}} = \dfrac{x \text{ g}}{250 \text{ ml}}$    $x = 20$ g

To prepare a 15% w/w solution of sodium bicarbonate in a liquid with a specific gravity of 2:
1. Add 15 g sodium bicarbonate to a flask.
2. Since 100 g solution is desired:

$$\begin{array}{r} 100 \text{ g solution} \\ -\ 15 \text{ g solute} \\ \hline 85 \text{ g diluent needed} \end{array}$$

3. Since specific gravity is 2 (1 ml weighs 2 g), how many milliliters will provide the desired 85 g?

$$\frac{1 \text{ ml}}{2 \text{ g}} = \frac{x \text{ ml}}{85 \text{ g}} \quad x = 42.5 \text{ ml}$$

4. Add 42.5 ml of liquid and dissolve.

To prepare 100 ml of a 50% w/v solution of formic acid (concentrated formic acid: specific gravity 1.2, 90.5% w/w):

1. 50% w/v = $\dfrac{50 \text{ g}}{100 \text{ ml}}$

How much of the liquid stock formic acid must be used to obtain the required 50 g?

2. Since specific gravity is 1.2, 1 ml of formic acid weighs 1.2 g, of which 90.5% is formic acid.

$$\frac{1.2 \text{ g}}{1 \text{ ml}} \times 0.905 = 1.09 \text{ g formic acid per milliliter}$$

3. Each milliliter of concentrated acid actually contains 1.09 g.

$$\frac{1 \text{ ml}}{1.09 \text{ g}} = \frac{x \text{ ml}}{50 \text{ g}} \quad x = 45.9 \text{ ml}$$

4. To prepare solution:
   a. To a 100 ml volumetric flask, add some distilled water.
   b. Add 48.9 ml concentrated formic acid.
   c. Dilute to 100 ml with distilled water.

## Molar (M) solutions

The molecular weight of a substance expressed in grams is called a mole (mol). A mole is also known as a gram-molecular weight.

To prepare 1 liter of a 1 molar solution of potassium hydroxide (KOH):

1. $1 \text{ M} = \dfrac{1 \text{ mol KOH}}{\text{Liter of solution}}$ (Atomic weight: $\begin{array}{ccc} \text{K} & \text{O} & \text{H} \\ 39 + 16 + 1 \end{array} = 56$)

2. $1 \text{ mol KOH} \times \dfrac{56 \text{ g}}{\text{Mole}} = 56 \text{ g}$

3. To a 1-liter volumetric flask, add 56 g KOH, dissolve in distilled water, and dilute to 1 liter.

To prepare 2 liters of a 0.5 M solution of potassium chloride (KCl):

1. $\dfrac{0.5 \text{ mol}}{\text{Liter}} \times 2 \text{ liters} \times \dfrac{74.5 \text{ g}}{\text{Mole}} = 74.5 \text{ g}$ (Atomic weight: $\begin{array}{cc} \text{K} & \text{Cl} \\ 39 + 35.5 \end{array} = 74.5$)

2. To a 2-liter volumetric flask, add 74.5 g KCl, dissolve in distilled water, and dilute to 2 liters.

How many millimoles (mmol) sodium hydroxide (NaOH) are contained in 50 ml of a 3 M solution?

1. $1 \text{ M} = \dfrac{1 \text{ mmol solute}}{\text{Milliliter solution}}$

2. $3 \text{ M} = \dfrac{3 \text{ mmol NaOH}}{\text{Milliliter solution}}$

3. $\dfrac{3 \text{ mmol}}{\text{Milliliter}} \times 50 \text{ ml} = 150 \text{ mmol}$

A solution contains 80.4 g NaOH in 600 ml of solution. What is its molarity? (Moles per liter must be found.)

1. Convert grams to moles and milliliters to liters:

$$\frac{80.4 \text{ g}}{600 \text{ ml}} \times \frac{1000 \text{ ml}}{\text{Liter}} \times \frac{1 \text{ mol}}{40 \text{ g}}$$

2. 3.35 mol per liter = 3.4 M

## Molal (mol/kg) solutions

A molal solution contains 1 mol of solute in 1000 g (1 kg) of solvent.

To prepare about 1 liter of a 1 molal aqueous solution of sulfuric acid ($H_2SO_4$) from concentrated $H_2SO_4$:

1. $1 \text{ molal} = \dfrac{1 \text{ mol } H_2SO_4}{1 \text{ kg solvent}}$

2. $\dfrac{1 \text{ ml}}{1.84 \times 0.98 \text{ g } H_2SO_4} \times \dfrac{98 \text{ g}}{\text{Mole}} = 54.3 \text{ ml per mole}$

3. 1 kg distilled water is needed.

## Normal (N) solutions

An equivalent is the quantity of a substance that will replace or react with 1.008 g (one atom) of hydrogen. When the weight of 1 eq is expressed in grams, it is called a gram-equivalent weight. A normal solution contains 1 gram-equivalent weight in 1 liter of solution.

How many grams of sodium chloride (NaCl) are needed to prepare 1 liter of a 1 N solution?　(Atomic weights: $\underset{23}{\text{Na}} + \underset{35.5}{\text{Cl}} = 58.5$)

1. Since 1 mol of NaCl will react with one replaceable hydrogen, 1 mol equals 1 eq.
2. The weight of 1 mol or 58.5 g is needed.

How many grams of phosphoric acid ($H_3PO_4$) are needed to prepare 1 liter of a 1 N solution? One mole contains three replaceable hydrogens:

$$\frac{1 \text{ mol}}{3 \text{ eq}} \times \frac{98 \text{ g}}{\text{Mole}} = 32.7 \text{ g/eq needed}$$

## Dilutions

Whenever a solution is diluted, its volume (V) is increased and its concentration (C) is decreased, but the total solute contained remains unchanged. Therefore two solutions of different volumes and of different concentrations can have the same amount of solute contained, for example:

$$\text{meq of solution no. 1} = \text{meq of solution no. 2}$$
$$V_1 \times C_1 = V_2 \times C_2$$

What volume of a 10% NaCl solution is required to prepare 500 ml of a 0.9% solution?

1. $V_1 \times C_1 = V_2 \times C_2$
2. $x \text{ ml} \times 10\% = 500 \text{ ml} \times 0.9\%$

3. $x = \dfrac{500 \times 0.9}{10} = 45 \text{ ml}$

36

## Conversion of units of concentration

To convert 2 N NaCl to percent concentration:

$$\frac{2 \text{ eq}}{1} \times \frac{58 \text{ g}}{1 \text{ eq}} \times \frac{1 \text{ liter}}{1000 \text{ ml}} \times 100 \text{ ml} = 11.6\%$$

To convert 1 N HCl to molarity:

$$\frac{1 \text{ eq}}{\text{liter}} \times \frac{1 \text{ mol}}{1 \text{ eq}} = \frac{1 \text{ mol}}{\text{Liter}} = 1 \text{ M}$$

To convert 4 M $H_3PO_4$ to normality:

$$4 \text{ M} \times 3 = 12 \text{ N or } \frac{4 \text{ mol}}{\text{Liter}} \times \frac{3 \text{ eq}}{\text{Mole}} \times \frac{12 \text{ eq}}{\text{Liter}} = 12 \text{ N}$$

## Temperature conversion

1. Kelvin = Centigrade + 273
2. Centigrade = 5/9(F−32)
3. Fahrenheit = (9/5C) + 32

*See worksheet, p. 99.*

## RADIOIMMUNOASSAY (RIA)

The integration of radiochemical techniques provides a more sensitive and specific method for measurement of extraordinarily small quantities of substances not measurable before by other techniques. The techniques of (RIA), which now have been applied to numerous substances of various structures, developed as a result of the pioneering work of Yalow and Berson. In 1960 they described a procedure for the determination of plasma insulin.

The basic principles of RIA utilize the reaction between antigen and antibody. One of the basic characteristics of antibodies and the reactions they enter into is their specificity. An antibody will react with the antigen for which it is specific and will not cross-react with similar-type antigens.

The antibodies needed in performing an RIA procedure are generally produced by injecting animals with the antigen to which the antibodies are desired. The animals will then develop these antibodies as part of their natural immune response. In turn, the serum derived from these animals is used as the antibody source.

The most common radioactive labels employed in RIA to date are $^{125}I$, $^{131}I$, and $^{3}H$. $^{125}I$ is usually the label of choice in commercially available products. Most peptides contain tyrosine, and the introduction of iodine into a tyrosine residue is easily facilitated. $^{125}I$ is a gamma energy-emitting isotope for which a solid crystal well counter is utilized.

The underlying mechanism for the assay involves competition between radioactively labeled and unlabeled antigens for a limited number of combining sites on the antibody. The reaction takes place in the presence of excess antigen. At equilibrium the ratio of antibody-bound labeled antigen to bound unlabeled antigen is proportional to the ratio of the initial concentrations of the two anti-

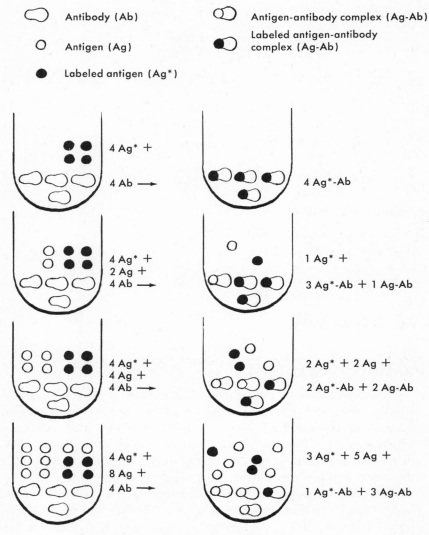

**Fig. 7-1.** Principle of radioimmunoassay.

genic species. The amount of bound label decreases as the concentration of unlabeled antigen increases.

Competitive binding assays utilize the same basic principles of isotope dilution and competitive reaction for a specific binding site. The major difference between competitive binding radioassay and RIAs is that competitive binding radioassays use substances other than antibodies as the binding agents.

## SPECTROPHOTOMETRY

PRINCIPLE: Chemical substances absorb ultraviolet and visible radiation because of the presence of certain chemical groups within the molecular system. This absorption is characteristic of the various functional groups that comprise the molecule, and therefore the absorption spectrum can be used as a means of identifying the type of substance present. The function of the spectrophotometer is to establish the degree of interaction between the sample and a beam of light at a particular wavelength. Several major components are essential to a spectrophotometer: a source of radiation, a monochromator that separates the radiation according to wavelength, a detector that converts the optical beam into an electrical signal, an electronic system to amplify and process the detection output, and a read-out device.

MATERIALS: Coleman Model 6/20A Junior IIA Spectrophotometer

PROCEDURE: Operation of the Coleman Junior is as follows:

1. Turn FUNCTION selector to %T.
2. Insert a cuvette adapter in cuvette well to block light path. Place light shield over cuvette well to prevent outside light from entering instrument.
3. Adjust ZERO control so scale indicates exactly 0.0%T.
4. Insert a cuvette containing reference material (blank) into cuvette well. Replace light shield over well.
5. Turn FUNCTION selector to %T or A, as desired.
6. Using SCALE ADJUSTER large and small knobs, set scale at exactly 100.0%T or 0.00 A.
7. Replace reference cuvette with a cuvette containing sample material. Read value of sample in terms of %T or A. NOTE: FUNCTION selector may be changed from %T to A (or A to %T) without re-referencing.

CALCULATIONS: The relationship between absorbance (A) and percent transmittance (%T) is as follows:

$$A = 2 - \log\%T$$

The law that forms the basis of spectrophotometry is the Beer-Lambert law or Beer's law. This is expressed as

$$A = Kcl$$

where $A$ is the absorbance, $K$ is a mathematical constant, $c$ is the molar concentration of the substance, and $l$ is the length of the cuvette in centimeters through which the light travels. For an analysis to be valid, it must follow Beer's law. This can be determined by plotting the log%T or absorbance against the concentration. If Beer's law is followed, the result of both graphs will be a straight line.

## RENAL DISEASES

The kidneys are bean-shaped structures situated in the posterior part of the abdominal cavity. The kidney has multiple functions, but the most important is its role in the body metabolism in the formation of urine. This entails not only the excretion of waste products from the blood but also the provision for the preservation of essential solutes and regulation of hydration and electrolyte balance.

Renal diseases make up a major portion of the total number of diseases. Disease may attack persons of any age. Some diseases will attack several parts of the kidneys at once; other diseases only attack one part. All lesions in renal diseases lead to derangements in the blood chemistry, cause pain in the renal region, alter the urinary output, and may result in signs and symptoms of renal insufficiency and azotemia. Azotemia is the presence of urea or other nitrogenous bodies in the blood.

Acute renal failure is characterized by a severe oliguric or anuric phase followed by a diuretic phase. Acute pyelonephritis, acute glomerulitis, and renal cortical necrosis are diseases that can lead to acute renal failure.

Glomerulonephritis is an inflammatory condition affecting the glomeruli of the kidney. As one of the most common types of kidney disease, it may be due to hypersensitivity, embolization, or bacteria. Acute glomerulonephritis seems to be related to an infection that has preceded it. *Streptococcus* is the most common causative bacterial agent. The infectious diseases that may precede the attack are tonsillitis, sore throat, rheumatic fever, or scarlet fever. Hematuria, pyuria, albuminuria, and casts are classic findings.

Pyelonephritis is the most common single type of renal disease. Obstruction somewhere in the urinary tract is associated with this disease. Obstructions predispose to infection, and the bacteria (usually *Escherichia coli*) are carried in the bloodstream to the kidney. Symptoms include sudden pain in the back, chills, fever, nausea, vomiting, and dysuria.

Another common disease of the kidney caused by obstruction is hydronephrosis. Urinary calculi are frequently the cause of the obstruction as well as carcinomas in the ureters or bladder.

Because the kidney is such a complex organ, there are a number of laboratory tests that can be employed in the diagnosis of kidney diseases. These kidney function tests can be divided into three groups: (1) those measuring glomerular filtration, (2) those measuring tubular function, and (3) those measuring renal blood flow. Any action that results in alteration or destruction of kidney tissue is critical because of the accumulation of toxic materials in the blood. Chemical tests are used to determine the nature and extent of this damage.

## Serum creatinine

PRINCIPLE: Creatinine reacts with alkaline picrate solution to give a red color (the so-called Jaffe reaction). The color reaction is not specific for creatinine; it is given by other substances in blood. However, the chromogenic material measured in normal plasma by this reaction is, according to the best evidence, 90% to 95% creatinine. A large part of the chromogenic material in the cells is not creatinine. Consequently the analysis is preferably made on serum.

REAGENTS:

1. Picric acid, 0.040 M: 10.17 g reagent grade picric acid (containing 10% to 12% added water), made up to 1 liter with distilled water. Place in 37° C water bath to bring picric acid into solution. Exact standardization of the acid is not required. Solution is stable at room temperature but should be protected from sunlight.
2. Sodium hydroxide 10% (w/v): dissolve 100 g sodium hydroxide in distilled water and dilute to 1000 ml.
3. Sulfuric acid, 0.058 N: dilute 1.75 ml of concentrated sulfuric acid to 1 liter in a volumetric flask with distilled water. Mix well.
4. Sodium tungstate 7% (w/v): dissolve 70 g reagent grade sodium tungstate ($Na_2WO_4 \cdot 2H_2O$) in water and dilute to volume in a 1 liter volumetric flask. This solution is stable indefinitely.
5. Stock creatinine standard; Harleco creatinine standard, No. 2412.

**40**

6. Working standard: transfer 0.5 ml stock standard into a 100 ml volumetric flask. Dilute to volume with distilled water. Make up fresh each time. This solution equals 5 mg/dl.

PROCEDURE:

1. Serum protein-free filtrate: into a 15 ml centrifuge tube measure the following:
   a. Add 1.0 ml serum to 8.0 ml 0.058 N sulfuric acid and mix by swirling.
   b. Add 1.0 ml 7% w/v sodium tungstate, cover with parafilm and shake vigorously.
   c. Centrifuge for 10 min at 2000 rpm; supernatant must be clear.
2. Serum creatinine: into four cuvettes place the following:
   a. Blank: 5.0 ml of distilled water and 2.5 ml of alkaline picrate solution (prepare freshly by adding 1 volume of 10% sodium hydroxide to 5 volumes of 1% picric acid)
   b. Standard: 5.0 ml working creatinine solution and 2.5 ml alkaline picrate solution
   c. Control: 5.0 ml protein-free filtrate of control serum and 2.5 ml alkaline picrate solution
   d. Unknown: 5.0 ml protein-free filtrate of unknown serum and 2.5 ml alkaline picrate solution
3. Cover tubes with parafilm and mix by inversion. Put in a dark place and read in 10 min at 540 nm. Read all three tubes against reagent blank.

CALCULATIONS:

$$\frac{\text{Value of standard}}{\text{Reading of standard}} \times \text{Reading of control or unknown} =$$

$$\text{Value of control or unknown in mg/dl}$$

NORMAL VALUE: 0.7 to 1.2 mg/dl.

*See worksheet, p. 101.*

## Blood urea nitrogen (BUN) (Hyland)

PRINCIPLE: Ammonia produced by the action of urease on urea, preformed ammonia, or ammonia derived from Kjeldahl digestion is determined by the Hyland phenate-hypochlorite method (modified Berthelot reaction). Ammonia reacts with phenol and sodium hypochlorite in the presence of a sodium nitroprusside catalyst to form indophenol, which exhibits a stable blue color, the intensity of which is directly proportional to the ammonia concentration. The color reaction is highly sensitive, reproducible, and requires only small specimen volumes. Therefore no deproteinization is required for the urea nitrogen determination.

REAGENTS: Use ammonia-free distilled water for preparation of reagents. Carefully clean glassware and pipettes (soak in cold dichromate cleaning solution

**41**

and rinse at least six times with distilled water) and avoid contamination with saliva.

1. Buffered urease, dried (in ethylenediamine tetraacetic acid [EDTA]), 30 units: reconstitute by adding 20 ml distilled water to vial. Reconstituted urease is stable for 1 month when stored between 2° and 8°C. Aliquots of freshly reconstituted reagent may be stored frozen for an indefinite period.

2. Phenol color reagent (phenol with sodium nitroprusside catalyst), 5 g:
   a. Warm vial by immersing in hot water a few minutes to liquefy phenol.
   b. Transfer contents of vial to a 100 ml container; rinse vial with distilled water to complete transfer; dilute to 100 ml and label. *Do not pipette by mouth: avoid contact with skin.*
   c. Store in amber glass or plastic between 2° and 8°C. This solution is stable for at least 6 months when protected from light.

3. Alkali-hypochlorite reagent (sodium hydroxide and sodium hypochlorite), 14 ml:
   a. Remove cap and puncture seal; be sure punctured opening is clear and then squeeze repeatedly to transfer contents. Dilute to 100 ml with distilled water.
   b. Store in glass or plastic containers between 2° and 8°C. This solution is stable for at least 6 months.

4. Nitrogen standard, 15 mg/100 ml (ammonium sulfate, 70.7 mg/100 ml), 3.5 ml: store between 2° and 8°C.

PROCEDURE: The test may be performed on plasma, serum, or diluted urine. Use ammonia-free distilled water throughout.

1. Pipette 0.2 ml reconstituted urease into each of three 10 ml test tubes (one for the test, one to serve as a reagent blank, and one to serve as a standard).

2. To sample tube add 0.020 ml specimen (plasma, serum, or 1:100 diluted urine). A calibrated Sahli hemoglobin pipette (20 cu mm) is convenient for this purpose. Use "washout" procedure. To blank add 0.020 ml distilled water. To standard add 0.020 ml nitrogen standard (15 mg/dl).

3. Incubate tubes in a heating block or water bath
   a. At room temperature (25°C) for at least 30 min
   b. Or at 37°C for at least 15 min
   c. Or at 50°C for 4 to 6 min

4. Add 1.0 ml reconstituted phenol color reagent and 1.0 ml diluted alkali-hypochlorite reagent to each tube in order specified. Promptly mix contents of each tube by inverting against pieces of inert material such as Saran Wrap (Dow) or Parafilm (Marathon).

5. Incubate in a water bath or heating block
   a. At room temperature (25°C) for at least 30 min
   b. Or at 37°C for at least 15 min
   c. Or at 50°C to 55°C for 5 to 7 min

6. Add 8 ml distilled water to each tube. Mix thoroughly by inversion.

7. Absorbance (A) reading
   a. Read absorbance of specimen using blank to zero photometer. Blank

absorbance should not exceed 0.14 at 630 nm (m$\mu$)—using a 1 cm cell in a spectrophotometer—when read against water. If blank reading is greater, distilled water and reagents have become contaminated with ammonia or ammonium salts, or reagents have aged too long.

b. Read absorbance of specimen. Peak absorbance is near 630 nm. However, any wavelength between 500 and 660 nm can be used (for example, Klett filter No. 66). If color is too intense to be read at 630 nm, use lower wavelength or dilute unknown and blank with distilled water and multiply final answer by dilution factor.

CALCULATIONS: The absorbance of the unknown is directly proportional to the ammonia nitrogen concentration:

$$\frac{\text{Value of standard}}{\text{Reading of standard}} \times \text{Reading of control or unknown} =$$

Value of control or unknown in mg/dl

INTERPRETATION:

| Specimen | Concentration |
|---|---|
| Plasma or serum | 8 to 20 mg/dl |
| Urine | 9 to 16 g/24 hr |

*See worksheet, p. 103.*

*See worksheet, p. 103.*

## CARBOHYDRATE METABOLISM

Carbohydrates supply the majority of energy needed by the body. The process of carbohydrate utilization by cells is called *catabolism*. The metabolism of carbohydrates is interrelated with that of fat and protein, since when carbohydrate stores are inadequate, the fats and proteins are mobilized as supplementary energy or fuel sources.

The most important carbohydrate is glucose, and metabolism starts with its transport through the cell membranes. Immediately following a meal, glucose can pass from the small intestine into the blood without being changed as the complex carbohydrates must be. Next a process called *glycogenesis* takes place where the temporary excess of carbohydrates is changed into glycogen. This is done by the liver cell in the presence of insulin. Glycogen is then stored in the liver and skeletal muscles until it is needed. At that time it is changed back into glucose by a process called *glycogenolysis*. When glucose is inadequate to meet the demands of the body, a process called *gluconeogenesis* takes place. In the process glucose is produced from fats or amino acids and then diffuses out of the liver cell into the blood. When blood glucose remains higher than normal after glycogenesis and catabolism in the presence of adequate insulin levels, the excess glucose is converted into fat by the liver cells and is then stored as adipose tissue.

The most common disease related to carbohydrate metabolism is diabetes mellitus. Diabetes means a "running through," and mellitus means "sweet."

Diabetes mellitus is thus a condition in which there is an excessive outpouring of urine containing sugar. The disease is characterized by insufficient levels of active insulin, and the body is not able to utilize carbohydrates and fats. We do not know the essential cause of diabetes, but there is a strong hereditary predisposition with evidence now accumulating that it is transferred by a recessive gene. The disease may develop from a faulty production of insulin by the pancreas, increased destruction of insulin during metabolism, faulty utilization of insulin, or increased tissue requirements for insulin to maintain normal carbohydrate metabolism. In any case there is not enough insulin produced, or the body does not make proper use of it. The result is a buildup of blood sugar (hyperglycemia) and thus glucose in the urine (glycosuria).

There are two types of diabetes: juvenile and adult. Juvenile diabetes occurs in patients under 25 years of age and has an onset at the average age of 11 years. The adult type develops in mainly obese people over 40 years of age. In this type the beta cells of the pancreas are incapable of releasing sufficient insulin to maintain a normal glucose level.

The chief signs and symptoms of untreated diabetes are polyuria (excessive urination), glycosuria (sugar in the urine), hyperglycemia (high blood sugar), polydipsia (excessive thirst), polyphagia (excessive appetite), and loss of weight and strength. Polyuria develops because large amounts of water are mobilized from the tissues to dilute the sugar brought to the kidneys, so that it can be eliminated. The tissues are dehydrated by the excessive loss of water, and this causes the polydipsia. When the patient is unable to utilize the glucose, he becomes weak, and this in turn causes polyphagia.

The complications of diabetes mellitus usually involve the vascular, endocrine, and nervous systems, but other systems can also be affected.

Arteriosclerosis, a hardening of the arteries, is likely to be more progressive and appear at an earlier age in diabetics as compared to nondiabetics. Coronary artery disease may also develop. The retina may be damaged, and blindness occurs. Kidney symptoms are edema, albuminuria, hypertension, and even renal failure. Because of the devitalization of the tissues by the sugar stored in them, gangrene can occur in the lower extremities. Diabetics have an increased susceptibility to infection. When the peripheral nerves are involved, there may be paresthesia (abnormal sensation), muscular weakness, and loss of reflexes.

Insulin is not a cure for diabetes, but it gives the overworked islets of Langerhans a much-needed rest. As a result, they may regain to some extent the power of attending to the carbohydrate needs of the body. Now as the result of insulin treatment, most patients do not die of diabetes but of complications and infections.

Hypoglycemia is a condition in which the blood sugar falls below normal levels. It can occur as a result of overdose of insulin but is usually the result of factors that reduce insulin, such as inadequate food intake or long delay in eating following an insulin injection, vigorous exercise with increased energy requirements, or vomiting and diarrhea that interferes with food absorption. Hyperinsulinism may aslo be caused by the presence of a tumor in the islets, which may be a benign adenoma or a carcinoma. The patient suffers from attacks of faintness of increasing severity, convulsions, and loss of consciousness.

Diagnostic aids in detecting carbohydrate disorders are urine sugar, blood sugar, and insulin levels. The blood sugar determination may be made on fasting blood samples or postprandial blood samples. Many times a glucose tolerance test is necessary to detect mild or very early cases.

## Enzymatic test for glucose (Trinder method)

PRINCIPLE: This test is based on the following reactions:

$$\text{Glucose} + O_2 + H_2O + GOD \rightarrow \text{Gluconic acid} + \text{Hydrogen peroxide}$$

$$\text{Hydrogen peroxide} + \text{Hydrogen donor dye (colorless)} + POD \rightarrow$$
$$\text{Hydrogen donor dye (green)} + 2H_2O$$

Glucose in the urine reacts with glucose oxidase (GOD) in aqueous solution to form gluconic acid and hydrogen peroxide. The hydrogen peroxide in the presence of peroxidase (POD) oxidizes a colorless donor dye, thus forming a green dye.

SPECIMEN: Use serum or plasma free of hemolysis.

REAGENTS:

1. To prepare working solution, dilute contents of one bottle BMC (Boehringer Mannheim Co.) with distilled or deionized water as follows:
   a. 150 ml water for each bottle of Cat. No. 15754
   b. 300 ml (2 bottles) water for each bottle of Cat. No. 15755
   c. 1000 ml (3 bottles) water for each bottle of Cat No. 15756
2. Reconstituted reagent is stable for 6 weeks at 4°C.
3. Store in amber bottle.

PROCEDURE:

1. Wavelength: 580 to 660 nm; temperature: room temperature.
2. Bring working solution to room temperature. Each series of tests requires one blank assay and one standard serum.
3. Pipette into test tubes:

|  | Blank | Specimen |
| --- | --- | --- |
| a. Deionized or distilled water | 0.02 ml | — |
| b. Serum or plasma | — | 0.02 ml |
| c. Working solution | 5.0 ml | 5.0 ml |

4. Mix and allow to stand at room temperature. Avoid exposure of tubes to direct sunlight. After 25 to 50 min, during which end-color is stable, transfer reaction mixture into cuvette and record absorbance of specimen reaction against zeroed blank.

CALCULATIONS:

$$\frac{\text{Value of standard}}{\text{Reading of standard}} \times \text{Reading of control or unknown} =$$
$$\text{Value of control or unknown in mg/dl}$$

NORMAL VALUE: Fasting: 70 to 105 mg/dl.

*See worksheet, p. 105.*

**Ortho-toluidine (o-Toluidine) glucose**

PRINCIPLE:

1. Label four Pyrex tubes as follows and add indicated solution and serums:

|  | Reagent blank | Standard | Control | Unknown |
|---|---|---|---|---|
| Distilled water | 0.1 ml | — | — | — |
| Glucose standard | — | 0.1 ml | — | — |
| Control | — | — | 0.1 ml | — |
| Patient's serum | — | — | — | 0.1 ml |
| o-Toluidine reagent | 5.0 ml | 5.0 ml | 5.0 ml | 5.0 ml |

2. Mix each tube by lateral shaking and place in boiling water bath for exactly 10 min. Remove and place in beaker of cold water to cool to room temperature (approximately 10 min).
3. Pour each into respectively labeled Coleman Jr. tubes. Read each in a spectrophotometer at 620 nm, setting instrument at zero using reagent blank, read within 30 min.

CALCULATIONS:

$$\frac{\text{Value of standard}}{\text{Reading of standard}} \times \text{Reading of control or unknown} =$$

$$\text{Value of control or unknown in mg/dl}$$

NORMAL VALUE: Fasting: 70 to 110 mg/dl.

*See worksheet, p. 107.*

## THE LIVER

The liver is the largest and, from a metabolic standpoint, the most complex internal organ in the body. Hepatic diseases are characterized by metabolic disturbances, and detection of these disturbances can serve as a diagnostic aid. Because the liver performs so many diverse metabolic functions, a great many tests of its functions have been devised, some of which are not clinically practicable.

The functions of the liver may be classified in four major groups:

1. Circulatory functions: transfer of blood from portal to systemic circulation activity of its reticuloendothelial system in immune mechanisms; blood storage
2. Excretory functions: bile formation and excretion of bile into the intestine; secretion in the bile of products emanating from the liver parenchymal cells
3. Metabolic functions: carbohydrate, lipid, protein, vitamin and mineral metabolism, and heat production
4. Protective functions and detoxification: Kupffer cell activity in removing foreign bodies from the blood (phagocytosis); detoxification by conjugation, methylation, oxidation, and reduction

## Liver function tests

The multiplicity and complexity of liver functions prevent us from using one test to tell us about the disburbances of its function. Perhaps this is the reason that tests are continually changing in number and variety. It may be said that tests for liver function fall into two main groups:

1. Differential diagnosis of the various types of jaundice
2. Estimation of liver damage in the absence of jaundice

In estimating liver damage the most sensitive tests are serum bilirubin, tests for bile pigments in the urine, and the Bromsulphalein (BŚP) excretion test, which is probably the best test for estimating the total functioning mass of hepatic tissue in the nonjaundiced patient. It has also been found that turbidity tests such as the thymol turbidity test, which involves the gamma globulin level in the serum, may be valuable in testing the course of liver diseases. In addition, liver enzymes that enter the blood have provided valuable information. Of these, glutamic oxaloacetic transaminase, glutamic pyruvic transaminase, and alkaline phosphatase are the most commonly determined.

## Diseases of the liver

**Hepatitis.** The term hepatitis signifies inflammation of the liver. This reaction to irritation is shown by necrosis of the hepatic cells. If the injury is only slight, the transient dead cells are quickly removed and replaced by new liver cells. When the injury is severe and prolonged, there is a proliferation of fibroblasts resulting in fibrosis, which in the liver is known as cirrhosis.

There are three main groups of hepatitis or hepatic necrosis: viral, toxic, and deficiency.

*Viral hepatitis.* Viral hepatitis is an acute diffuse hepatic necrosis that occurs both in sporadic and epidemic form. The sporadic form is mild and shows itself as a transient attack of jaundice. The epidemic form is more severe. The virus is excreted in the stools and is transmitted by oral ingestion of infected material. There are two types of viral hepatitis caused by different but related viruses with practically identical clinical pictures: infectious hepatitis and serum or syringe hepatitis. Serum hepatitis is usually transmitted by the intravenous injection of human serum or by a syringe or needle that has become infected by such serum.

Liver lesions vary greatly in severity. In the exceptional fulminating case the necrotic liver is extremely soft, bright yellow in color, and may lose half of its weight in the course of a week. This is known as acute yellow atrophy and is fatal. However, usually there is complete recovery from viral hepatitis, but in an occasional case cirrhosis may develop.

The symptoms of hepatitis also vary. In the most severe cases (acute yellow atrophy) the onset is sudden and the course acute, including vomiting, jaundice, bile in the urine, delirium, coma, and death. In the more ordinary well-developed case there is loss of appetite (anorexia), fever, jaundice, bile in the urine, and fatigue.

*Toxic hepatitis.* Toxic hepatitis is a necrosis of the liver caused by drugs and by chemicals used in technical processes, particularly carbon tetrachloride.

*Deficiency hepatitis.* Relatively little is known about deficiency hepatitis in humans. Most of the knowledge of this disease is from feeding experiments on laboratory animals. When kept on a prolonged diet deficient in protein and other various food factors, the liver cells first become greatly distended with fat and then undergo necrosis and cirrhosis. In chronic alcoholism the diet is nearly always deficient in the protective food substances. Gastritis impairs the appetite of the chronic alcoholic, and calories are supplied by the alcohol, which takes the place of food. In the African Bantu, dietary deficiency is responsible for the widespread prevalence of cirrhosis, which is frequently associated with carcinoma. *Kwashiorkor*, an African term meaning "red boy," is a nutritional disease prevalent in children as well as adults. In this disease there is a lesion in the liver with an extreme degree of fatty infiltration and ensuing cirrhosis.

**Cirrhosis.** Cirrhosis is a progressive chronic destruction, diffuse in extent, and accompanied by fibrosis. The liver assumes a characteristic appearance: in the early stages it is enlarged, but as the disease progresses the liver becomes smaller and the surface becomes nodular due to extensive scarring by fibrous tissue. The surface becomes covered with little knobs of tissue and is sometimes called a "hobnailed" liver.

Obstruction to the portal vein is the most important effect of cirrhosis. The pathways through which blood passes through the liver are distorted and obliterated by the scarring and tissue destruction, so that blood is backed up and collects in the portal vein and its branches. Jaundice may develop in the late stages of cirrhosis, owing to interference with the excretion of bile, which accumulates in the blood and tinges the skin, the whites of the eyes, and the tissues.

**Jaundice or icterus.** Jaundice is a coloration of the skin by bile pigment in the blood. The color varies from pale yellow to deep orange or even green. The pigment, bilirubin, is a breakdown product of red blood cells. This breakdown takes place in the reticuloendothelial system (lymph nodes, spleen, and so on) and is then excreted by the liver, passing first by the bile ducts to the gallbladder and then along the common bile duct to the duodenum.

There are three ways in which bilirubin may accumulate in excess in the blood and so give rise to jaundice.

*Obstructive jaundice.* The liver may excrete bile normally, but it may be unable to escape into the duodenum because of some obstruction. The two most common causes of obstruction are gallstones lodged in the common bile duct and carcinoma of the head of the pancreas, which blocks the opening of the duct into the duodenum. In these instances the bile accumulates in the liver and is reabsorbed into the blood. The urine is colored with bile, and since no bile reaches the intestine, the stools are extremely pale and are described as clay-colored.

*Hepatic jaundice.* When the liver is extensively damaged, as in hepatitis, it is unable to excrete the bilirubin brought to it, which therefore accumulates in the blood.

*Hemolytic jaundice.* Hemolytic jaundice is caused by abnormal breaking down of the red blood cells. If an extensive amount of blood is broken down, more bilirubin will be formed than can be excreted by the liver, so that it will remain in the blood. This condition is seen in extensive internal hemorrhage when the wrong type of blood is transfused and in congenital hemolytic anemia.

## Serum thymol turbidity

PRINCIPLE: Patients who have hepatitis demonstrate an increase in beta globulin in their serum. This increase in beta globulin will cause a turbidity when mixed with a thymol solution in barbiturate buffer. This turbidity is caused by a globulin-thymol-phospholipid complex.

REAGENTS:

1. Thymol tris buffer (Dade).
2. 0.85% saline: place 8.5 g Na Cl in a 1000 ml volumetric flask. Add distilled water to 1 liter mark.

PROCEDURE:

1. A blank and test are set up for each serum as follows:

|  | **Blank** | **Test** |
|---|---|---|
| Standard | 6.0 ml saline | 6.0 ml thymol buffer |
| Control | 6.0 ml saline | 6.0 ml thymol buffer |
| Unknown | 6.0 ml saline | 6.0 ml thymol buffer |

2. Add 0.1 ml of the respective sera to each of the blank test tubes.
3. Parafilm the tubes and mix by gentle inversion several times. Do not shake. Let stand at room temperature for 30 min. Read at 420 nm. Read each test against its appropriate blank.

CALCULATIONS:

$$\frac{\text{Value of standard}}{\text{Reading of standard}} \times \text{Reading of control or unknown} =$$
$$\text{Value of control or unknown in thymol turbidity units}$$

NORMAL VALUE: 0 to 5 units.

## Serum total bilirubin

PRINCIPLE: Serum bilirubin is coupled with diazotized sulfanilic acid to form azobilirubin. Total bilirubin represents the sum of the conjugated bilirubin glucuronides (direct) and the unconjugated bilirubin (indirect).

REAGENTS:

1. Absolute methyl alcohol.
2. 1.5% v/v hydrochloric acid.
3. Diazo reagent: crush one diazo tablet and dissolve in 50 ml of 1.5% v/v hydrochloric acid.

PROCEDURE:

1. Set up a standard, control, and unknown as follows:

|  | **Blank** | **Test** |
|---|---|---|
| Distilled water | 2.0 ml | 2.0 ml |
| Serum | 0.2 ml | 0.2 ml |
| 1.5% hydrochloric acid | 0.5 ml | — |
| Diazo reagent | — | 0.5 ml |

**49**

2. Mix by lateral shaking and add 2.5 ml methyl alcohol to both blank and test.
3. Cover tubes with parafilm and mix by gently inverting. Let stand 15 min. Read at 540 nm against respective blanks.

CALCULATIONS:

$$\frac{\text{Value of standard}}{\text{Reading of standard}} \times \text{Reading of control or unknown} =$$

$$\text{Value of control or unknown in mg/dl.}$$

NORMAL VALUE: 0.2 to 1.3 mg/dl.

*See worksheet, p. 109.*

## TOXICOLOGY

The incidence of poisoning, both accidental and suicidal, has increased to an alarming level in recent years. The high incidence of poisonings of all types has led most hospitals and clinical laboratories to recognize the need for laboratory services that give rapid and reliable information about the type and quantity of poison ingested by the patient.

The modern toxicologic specialist uses common as well as other more sophisticated tools of science in isolating, identifying, and quantitating toxic substances in biologic material. In addition, he should be in a position to interpret the laboratory results, advise as to treatment of the patient, or give an opinion as to the effect, if any, of the toxic substance on the condition of the patient.

In medicolegal cases (criminal poisonings or cases in which legal action may be necessary) special precautions are necessary in collecting, transporting, and storing specimens to ensure that loss, tampering, or contamination cannot occur. The specimens and other evidence must be in the custody of a responsible individual at all times to establish a proper chain of custody and to avoid legal objections during the presentation of evidence in court.

The costly and complex laboratory procedures together with the legal problems and inconveniences of court testimony have had the result that most clinical laboratory directors are reluctant even to contemplate the performance of toxicologic tests. Such considerations need not and indeed should not prevent clinical laboratories from carrying out those tests that are within the limitations of their personnel and facilities. The useful information gained can be rapidly communicated to the clinician, which results in more intelligent and faster treatment and possibly the saving of lives.

### Gases

**Carbon monoxide.** The most common of the gaseous poisons is carbon monoxide, which is the product of incomplete combustion of organic substances. It is present in manufactured gas in the free state when used as fuel for stoves, furnaces, and other appliances. Poorly ventilated or malfunctioning heating appliances are therefore frequently a cause of carbon monoxide poisoning.

Carbon monoxide combines with hemoglobin in an identical manner to that of oxygen, but the bond is about 210 times stronger. As a result, carbon monoxide is not readily displaced from hemoglobin, and accidental poisonings can occur even at low levels of carbon monoxide in the atmosphere with prolonged exposure. In some instances the carbon monoxide level in blood builds up slowly until toxic levels are reached.

Symptoms include headache, giddiness, vomiting, vertigo, loss of memory, fainting, collapse, paralysis, and unconsciousness. Skin color varies from normal to flushed, cyanotic, or uncommonly, cherry-pink.

Detection may be approached in two ways:

1. Release of the gas from the hemoglobin complex with subsequent direct or indirect measurement
2. Estimation of carboxyhemoglobin by its typical color or absorption bands

The first method can be carried out by gasometric techniques, gas chromatography, microdiffusion, or infrared spectrophotometry. The second method utilizes spectrophotometric or simple color comparison.

Regardless of the analytic method used, the specimen to be analyzed must contain hemoglobin.

Treatment includes treatment with oxygen. In a high oxygen tension the carbon monoxide is released from the hemoglobin.

## Volatile substances

This group of toxic compounds consists mainly of liquids that have boiling points of 100°C or lower. Members of this group include almost all types of chemical compounds, and many are solvents commonly used in industry or in household products.

**Ethyl alcohol.** Ethanol is the most common toxic substance involved in medicolegal cases. It not only is lethal in its own right but it also is commonly a contributing factor in accidents of all types. In the case of a patient brought to the hospital in a coma, the effects of alcohol, if any, must be ruled out in a differential diagnosis of the cause of coma.

Symptoms include central nervous system depression and gastric irritation, with nausea and vomiting. Other manifestations include hypoglycemia, convulsions, fever (104° to 108°F), and cerebral edema with severe headache. There are probably more published methods for the determination of ethanol in blood than for any other toxic substance. In general they can be divided into those methods that are simple but nonspecific, and those that are specific but complex. In any event the collecting of the sample is important. Prep the arm with soap and water.

In the enzymatic procedure, ethanol is oxidized in the presence of alcohol dehydrogenase (ADH) to acetaldehyde.

$$C-C-OH \xrightarrow{\quad ADH \quad} C-C\!\!\diagdown\!\!\begin{array}{c} O \\ H \end{array}$$

NAD   NADH
(colorless) (colored)
at 340 nm

Blood levels up to 10 mg/dl can be considered negative, since negative bloods may contain this amount of volatile reducing substances. With blood levels of 50 to 100 mg/dl, various signs of intoxication may be observed: flushing, slowing of reflexes, impairment of visual acuity, and so on (there is much individual variation in this regard). Above 100 mg/dl all individuals are under the influence of alcohol, and depression of the central nervous system is more apparent. With higher levels, central nervous system impairment is more pronounced, and true coma may appear at levels of 300 mg/dl. Death may occur with levels above 400 mg/dl.

Treatment is to remove unabsorbed alcohol by gastric lavage with tap water, maintain the airway and respiration, and keep the patient warm.

**Methyl alcohol.** Methanol is used in solvents in paints, varnishes, and paint removers. It is used alone as an antifreeze fluid and with ethanol and soap as a solid canned fuel. Poisonings are usually due to accidental ingestion by children or by alcoholics.

It is a central nervous system depressant, which produces specific damage to the retinal cells and metabolic acidosis; the minimum lethal dose is 30 to 60 ml. Symptoms include headache, nausea, abdominal pain, vomiting, dyspnea, and blindness. Examination reveals flush or cyanosis, excitement or depression, delirium, coma, and convulsions.

Methanol can be determined by a variety of methods, most of which involve measuring the color intensity after oxidation of methanol to formaldehyde with chromotropic acid. Gas chromatography is considered to be the best method.

Methanol is metabolized to fomaldehyde and formic acid. This accumulation of formic acid reduces the alkali reserve, causing a metabolic acidosis. In addition, necrosis of the pancreas and subsequent increases in serum amylase have been observed. Therefore, in addition to blood methanol levels, plasma, carbon dioxide, pH, serum amylase, and electrolyte studies are helpful. Treatment is twofold: first, treat the acidosis: second, administer ethanol to saturate the ADH system. Ethanol is the preferred substrate for this enzyme, and this would prevent the conversion of methanol to its toxic metabolites.

**Cyanide.** Cyanide inhibits cellular respirations because of its combination with important respiratory enzymes. This mechanism of action is the same whether cyanide is inhaled as a gas, hydrocyanic acid, or ingested as the potassium or sodium salt, or other combined forms. Since death follows quickly if sufficient cyanide is absorbed, the patient rarely survives long enough for treatment. Despite this fact, it is desirable to have a test for this poison available to confirm a suspected cyanide death.

The clinical combination of cyanosis, asphyxia, and the odor of bitter almonds on the breath is diagnostic. Respiration is first stimulated and later depressed. A marked drop in blood pressure may occur.

To treat, induce vomiting immediately with a finger down the patient's throat. Combat shock and give 100% oxygen by forced ventilation.

## Corrosives

This group includes those strong minerals, acids, or fixed alkalies that produce chemical burns on contact. There is no good test that can be carried out on blood, serum, or urine by which the type of acid or alkali can be detected and the ingested quantity estimated.

The only specimen that can be examined profitably is gastric contents. Frequently this specimen is not available unless the patient has vomited, since gastric lavage is contraindicated in this type of poisoning. If gastric contents are available, the pH should be measured.

## Metals

All metals are toxic if a sufficient quantity is absorbed. Generally they are not encountered in their toxic form in the elemental or free state, but rather in the form of salts.

**Arsenic.** Despite its reputation, arsenic is not a common poison. It is still a favorite homicidal poison, but homicidal poisonings are rare.

Symptoms include abdominal pain, difficulty in swallowing, persistent vomiting, diarrhea, urinary suppression, and skeletal muscle cramps. Later findings are severe thirst and shock.

Urine is the specimen of choice for determination of arsenic. It has a great affinity for sulfhydryl groups and thus combines readily with proteins. This results in the precipitation of proteins, producing gastrointestinal irritation and irreversible inhibition of important enzyme systems. It is also this affinity that is responsible for the rapid removal from the blood. The Reinsch test is used in determining the presence of heavy metals. Metallic copper in the presence of acid will reduce arsenic to the elemental form. The arsenic deposits on the copper as a visible, dark film.

Treatment is to induce vomiting.

**Lead.** Lead is still one of the most serious of metallic poisons, particularly in children who are exposed to paint and plaster containing lead. Severe poisoning in a child can cause lead encephalopathy, and those children who survive frequently show evidence of permanent central nervous system damage.

The demonstration of elevated lead level in blood or urine is necessary for a diagnosis of absorption of a lead compound.

Symptoms include metallic taste, irritability, apathy, anorexia, vomiting, abdominal colic, diarrhea, constipation, headache, leg cramps, black stools, stupor, oliguria, convulsions, and coma.

Usually atomic absorption spectroscopy is used for lead determinations. The clinical laboratory can perform two important functions that aid in the diagnosis of lead poisoning even if the lead analysis is done by others: (1) the specimens to be analyzed must be collected free of contamination and (2) other diagnostic tests can be done for screening purposes or for confirmation. These tests are based on the effects of lead on erythropoiesis. Although the precise mechanism is not understood, lead interferes in the biosynthesis of hemoglobin, which results in anemia. Two precursors of hemoglobin, delta-aminolevulinic acid and coproporphyrin, are markedly elevated in the urine.

## Nonmetals

The toxic nonmetals are usually encountered as compounds with other elements or as sodium and potassium salts. They are infrequently found in the free elemental form.

**Bromides.** Bromides are used in both organic and inorganic forms in medicine, chiefly for the purpose of sedation. These drugs may be abused or may be taken in overdosage accidentally.

Bromides are central nervous system depressants, and symptoms include anorexia, constipation, drowsiness, apathy, and hallucinations.

Methods for bromide ($Br^-$) measure free bromide only; the bromide anion readily displaces chloride from gold trichloride ($AuCl_3$), forming gold tribromide ($AuBr_3$). The resulting color is brown.

$$AuCl_3 + 3Br^- \rightarrow AuBr_3 + 3Cl^-$$

Treatment is to lavage copiously with saline to remove unabsorbed bromides and force fluids.

### Nonvolatile organic substances

This is the largest group of substances and includes most drugs and alkaloids. Analysis of this group includes extraction methods to separate the drug from the specimen. These are frequently not quantitative or may result in troublesome emulsions or may be pH dependent. Some drugs are rapidly metabolized, excreted, or bound to protein, which makes their detection difficult. Those drugs that are weak acids or bases are usually water soluble when they are in the form of salts. By reconverting the drug back to the free acid or base, it is made less water soluble but more soluble in solvents such as chloroform or ether. This property of organic acids and bases is used in separation and purification steps. By adjusting the pH of the aqueous phase and extracting with less polar immiscible solvents, separation is usually successful. Those drugs that are neutral are more difficult to extract and purify.

The advent of thin-layer chromatography has been a great help in detecting organic drugs in extracts of biologic material. Although the extraction technique may not be quantitative, the speed and sensitivity of thin-layer chromatography enables the extract to be easily screened for the presence or absence of certain drugs or groups of drugs.

**Alkaloids.** The alkaline group consists of the opium alkaloids (morphine, codeine, heroin), cocaine, methadone, Darvon, meperidine (Demerol), amphetamine, phenothiazines, Valium, Librium, and methaqualone. Since these doses are low, urine is the sample of choice.

*Opiates.* Heroin is the most prevalent representative of the opiate group. Drowsiness, lethargy, and constricted pupils during acute intoxication, and needle puncture wounds are the main diagnostic points. The individual with a heavy habit who cannot support it has a day divided into three stages: (1) a hustle to find the money for the drug, (2) a 3- to 6-hour period of euphoria while on the "high," and (3) a postdrug period of sickness. Withdawal symptoms are similar to a severe case of influenza. Five to ten hours after the last dose of heroin there is a craving for the drug, anxiety, restlessness, runny eyes and nose, sweating, aches and pains, nausea, and chills.

The control of the heroin addict's habit can be affected by the use of methadone treatment. Methadone, also a habituating drug, requires careful dispensing.

*Morphine.* Morphine acts primarily on the central nervous system, causing depression and narcosis. The manifestations of poisoning with morphine and its substitutes, heroin, meperidine, Darvon, and methadone are headache, nausea, excitement, convulsions, depression, pinpoint pupils, slow respirations, apnea, rapid and feeble pulse, shock, and coma.

54

**Acid-neutrals.** This group contains the barbiturates, salicylates, glutethimide, meprobamate, phenytoin (Dilantin), and Noludar. Almost all of these drugs can be associated with coma and are of prime importance in screening the comatose patient.

*Barbiturates.* In acid form, barbiturates are relatively water insoluble, but they are soluble in organic solvents. They can be extracted from blood or serum at physiologic pH values or from acidified urine by organic solvents. Shaking the organic solvent with dilute alkaline solution converts the free acid form of barbiturate into the aqueous phase, which is scanned using the ultraviolet spectrophotometer.

Proper interpretation of a blood or serum barbiturate level cannot be done unless the type of barbiturate present is known. For example, a 1 mg/dl level of phenobarbital is not too serious, but the same level of secobarbital is close to a lethal level.

Pharmacologically the barbiturates can be classified according to their duration of action.

1. Long acting: phenobarbital, barbital
2. Intermediate: amobarbital, butabarbital
3. Short: pentobarbital, secobarbital
4. Ultrashort: hexobarbital, pentothal

Temperature-programmed gas chromatography provides a solution to the problem of time in analysis. In this method the column temperature is increased linearly with time during the analysis of a sample. As the temperature is increased, the compounds are eluted as sharp symmetrical peaks in order of their molecular structure.

**Hallucinogenic drugs.** Hallucinogenic drugs produce dilated pupils, heightened reflexes, and marked anxiety. Still, no good test is available, since such a small quantity is actually present in the body. However, some RIA procedures are being developed for this purpose.

## Pill identification

Sometimes a patient will be accompanied to the emergency room with pills in his possession. It is helpful to be able to classify these drugs by simple spot tests, but in no way should this be identified as the causative agent without identifying it in the specimens drawn or obtained from the patient. It is merely an aid in guiding the analyst in his systematic approach to the unknown.

## Acid-neutral extraction

PRINCIPLE: Thin-layer chromatography (TLC) is a simple technique for the separation of drugs. Chromatography depends on the interaction of two different phases: a stationary phase and a moving phase. An adsorbent is coated on an inert carrier (stationary phase). The developing solvent (moving phase) flows through the adsorbent on which the sample has been placed. Migration of the sample occurs by capillary action when the two phases contact each other in a glass tank.

The acid-neutral drug group contains the barbiturates, salicylates, glutethimide, meprobamate, Dilantin, and methyprylon.

REAGENTS:

1. 0.1 M citric acid: dissolve 21.01 g citric acid in 1000 ml distilled water.
2. 0.2 M sodium phosphate: dissolve 2.76 g sodium phosphate in 100 ml distilled water.
3. Citrate buffer, pH 2.2: mix 980 ml 0.1 M citric acid solution with 20 ml 0.2 M sodium phosphate.
4. Chloroform, reagent grade
5. Ethyl acetate, reagent grade
6. Methanol, reagent grade
7. Ammonium hydroxide, concentrated reagent grade
8. 1% silver acetate in water
9. 0.02 M potassium permanganate in water: store in a dark bottle.

PROCEDURE:

1. Place 15 ml urine into a 50 ml glass-stoppered round bottom centrifuge tube.
2. Add 10 ml citrate buffer, pH 2.2.
3. Add 10 ml chloroform and stopper tightly.
4. Shake 5 min and then centrifuge at 2000 rpm for 5 min.
5. Carefully aspirate off the aqueous layer (top) and the interface disk with a vacuum aspirator and discard.
6. Pour chloroform layer into an evaporating dish, being careful not to get any buffer into dish.
7. Evaporate to dryness in a circulating oven between 50° to 60° C. When dry, wash down sides with few drops of chloroform to concentrate residue at bottom of dish. Evaporate to dryness. Extract is now ready for TLC.
8. Lay out and cut TLC plates. Put all lines and spots on plate very lightly with pencil. Do not break surface of silica gel.
9. Place minimum amount of methanol (50 $\mu$l) in evaporating dish. Carefully swirl to dissolve residue. Let solvent evaporate to 20 to 30 $\mu$l.
10. Take up sample in a 5 $\mu$l disposable pipette.
11. Carefully spot TLC plates with 1 to 2 $\mu$l at a time to keep spots as small as possible. Let spot dry between applications.
12. Repeat spotting procedure for standards that have been dissolved in methanol.
13. Start TLC plate developing. Solvent system is ethylacetate 42.5 ml, methanol 5 ml, concentrated ammonium hydroxide 2.5 ml. Allow solvents to equilibrate in tank for at least 30 min before plate is placed in chamber.
14. Let solvent front run to within 1 cm of top.
15. Remove plate and allow to dry.
16. Place plate in a fume hood and spray until completely wet with silver acetate solution.
17. Spray with potassium permanganate in hood.

INTERPRETATION: The barbiturates all turn chalky white when sprayed with silver acetate. Doriden and Dilantin will also turn white. After spraying with potassium permanganate, the secobarb will turn yellow. The other barbiturates will turn pink. Dilantin and Doriden will remain white. Compare standard R$_f$

values with unknown $R_f$ values (ratio of the rates of migration of the acid-neutral drugs to that of the solvent front).

## Alkaline extraction

PRINCIPLE: Urine is used for the detection of cocaine, Demerol, Darvon, codeine, morphine, amphetamine, methamphetamine, quinine, Quaalude, nicotine, and caffeine.

REAGENTS:

1. 0.3 N sodium hydroxide: dissolve 1.36 sodium hydroxide pellets in 100 ml distilled water.
2. Borate buffer, pH 9.5: mix 930 ml of saturated sodium borate solution with 70 ml of 0.3 N sodium hydroxide.
3. Chloroform-isopropyl alcohol: mix three parts chloroform to one part isopropyl alcohol (v/v). Mix 30 min before using.
4. Iodoplatinate spray: add 10 ml of 10% solution platinum chloride to 250 ml of 4% potassium iodide and diluted 500 ml with distilled water. Store in dark bottle in refrigerator.

PROCEDURE:

1. Place 15 ml urine into a 50 ml glass-stoppered round bottom centrifuge tube.
2. Add 10 ml borate buffer, pH 9.5.
3. Add 10 ml chloroform-isopropyl alcohol (3:1).
4. Stopper tightly and shake for 5 min.
5. Centrifuge at 2000 rpm for 5 min.
6. Aspirate off the aqueous phase (top) and any interface disk with a vacuum aspirator and discard.
7. Carefully pour chloroform phase into an evaporating dish, being careful to avoid getting any buffer into dish.
8. Add 2 drops hydrochloric acid into dish. (Amphetamines are volatile unless converted to stable salt.)
9. Evaporate to dryness in a circulating oven between 50° to 60° C. When dry, wash sides of dish with a few drops of chloroform to concentrate residue at bottom of dish. Evaporate to dryness. Extract is now ready for TLC.
10. Lay out and cut TLC plate. Put all lines and spots on plate very lightly with pencil. Do not break surface of silica gel.
11. Spot TLC plate with standards and unknowns as described in previous procedures.
12. Develop plate in ethylacetate solvent system.
13. After development, spray TLC plate with ninhydrin and heat at 100°C for 2 to 3 minutes.
14. Spray plate with iodoplatinate.

INTERPRETATION: After spraying with ninhydrin and heating, amphetamines will appear as pink spots. Alkaloids will appear as purplish black spots after spraying with iodoplatinate.

*See worksheet, p. 111.*

## LIPIDS

Lipids are defined as water-insoluble organic substances that are extractable by nonpolar solvents such as chloroform, ether, and benzene. The principal lipids found in human serum are cholesterol, phospholipids, fatty acids, and triglycerides.

During the last decade, investigators interested in the problem of lipid metabolism have amassed an impressive body of evidence linking qualitative as well as quantitative changes in serum lipid patterns to accelerated coronary disease.

It has been suggested that the sulfophospho-vanillin reaction for estimating total serum lipid is a useful screening procedure for detecting hyperlipidemia.

### Total serum lipids: phospho-vanillin reaction

PRINCIPLE: The unsaturated lipids react with sulfuric acid to produce a carbonium ion. Vanillin reacts with phosphoric acid to produce an aromatic phosphate ester. When mixed, the carbonium ion reacts with the activated carbonyl group of phospho-vanillin to produce a pink color.

SPECIMEN: Blood should be drawn after a 12- to 14-hour fast.

REAGENTS:

1. Concentrated sulfuric acid.
2. Phospho-vanillin reagent: 0.60 g vanillin is dissolved in 10 ml absolute ethanol before diluting to 100 ml with distilled water. This solution was mixed with 400 ml concentrated phosphoric acid with constant stirring. Store in dark bottle at room temperature.
3. Total lipid standard solution: 700 mg oleic acid and 300 mg stearic acid were dissolved in water, enough 1 N potassium hydroxide being added to bring acids into solution, and diluted to 100 ml with distilled water (1000 mg/dl).

PROCEDURE:

1. Mark Pyrex tubes as follows: Blank, standard, control, and unknown.
2. Place 0.02 ml standard, control, and unknown serum into appropriate tubes. Add nothing to the blank.
3. Add 0.4 ml concentrated sulfuric acid to all tubes.
4. Place tubes in boiling water bath for 10 min.
5. Remove and cool to room temperature.
6. Add 10 ml phospho-vanillin reagent to all tubes.
7. Stopper with parafilm and mix by inversion.
8. Let tubes stand at room temperature and read at 525 nm against the blank.

CALCULATIONS:

$$\frac{\text{Value of standard}}{\text{Reading of standard}} \times \text{Reading of control or unknown} =$$

$$\text{Value of control or unknown in mg/dl}$$

1. Subjects with serum total lipid values below 600 mg/dl have little, if any, likelihood of having an abnormal lipid pattern.
2. Subjects with values in the range of 600 to 650 mg/dl are most likely normal, but could possibly have a borderline abnormality.
3. Subjects between 650 to 700 mg/dl should be considered suspect and more immediate detailed analysis carried out.
4. Subjects with values over 700 mg/dl will rarely have normal lipid patterns.

*See worksheet, p. 113.*

# 8 Microbiology

## INFECTIOUS DISEASES

An infection is an invasion of the body by microorganisms or biologic agents that cause tissue damage and disease. These microorganisms (bacteria, viruses, rickettsiae, fungi, protozoa, or helminths) cause disease as an expression of their struggle to survive.

Man exists in a world crowded with microorganisms, but few of them cause harm. Many of these microorganisms are not capable of causing harm, and many coexist with man without injury to their host. Man has overcome some harmful effects through acquired immunity as a result of previous exposure. The body's defense mechanisms prevent the flora of the skin, mouth, and body openings and surfaces from gaining entrance to the vital internal tissues. Because man is now aware of the potentialities of certain microorganisms, he can be on guard against them. Some microorganisms are actually beneficial to man. *Escherichia coli*, flora of the intestinal tract, produces vitamin K, an antihemorrhagic factor necessary for the maintenance of health.

Infectious diseases have plagued man since early biblical times, the most written about being leprosy. The plague, cholera, smallpox, and typhus have also occurred in epidemics, taking many lives. Many of these diseases have been eradicated through recognition of causative agents and through methods of control. Following World War I (1918-1919) there occurred an estimated 500 million cases of influenza with 15 million fatalities. In 1957 a pandemic occurrence of Asian influenza resulted in fewer deaths. The acute respiratory viral infections, such as influenza, rarely cause death themselves. It is usually the result of secondary bacterial invaders such as staphylococcus, pneumococcus, and meningococcus. Through the use of antibiotics, bacterial infections and some viral infections have been brought under control. However, an ever increasing number of organisms are becoming resistant to these drugs.

There are several reasons why infectious diseases are not as prevalent in our modern world. First, extensive investigations in the discovery of the organisms responsible for disease have resulted in immunizations or vaccines for protection, for example, diphtheria, measles, and smallpox. Second, discovery of the transmittance of disease has led to eradication, as in the discovery that the mosquito transmits malaria and yellow fever. Third, awareness of proper sanitation procedures has helped to control many intestinal infections (typhoid fever, cholera, dysentery, hookworm) that are spread through human excreta. Even though there are still problems with influenza outbreaks, the use of influenza vaccine has weakened the epidemics. Most of the investigative work on infectious diseases is now centered on the study of the viruses. Much of this work is in the interest of controlling influenza, but more research investigating viruses as the cause of cancer is now underway.

As a class of microorganisms, viruses are very small and have a simple chemical composition. They consist of an outer protein coat and an inner core of information-laden nucleic acids. Although viruses have no innate metabolism and no viability outside of host cells, they remain inert in the environment. Once introduced into the body, they suddenly become viable and cause damage to tissues. When the virus gets inside the cell, it is capable of taking over the work of the cell and disrupting its normal activity. The host cells do have a protection mechanism in which they produce interferon, which is directed against the foreign nucleic acids and interferes with the reproduction of viruses inside the cell.

The communicable diseases, so-called contagious, are transferred by contact between an infected individual and a healthy person through different modes of transmittance. Most bacteria and viruses are fragile and die in the environment. They cannot survive under adverse circumstances, which is the reason for personal hygiene and sanitation.

Man may also contract infection from the lower animals, especially through his close contact with domestic animals. To mention just a few, from horses he may contract glanders; from dogs, rabies or *Echinococcus* cysts; from cattle, undulant fever, anthrax, or tuberculosis; from hogs, ringworm; and from parrots, psittacosis. In the environment there are also rats, mice, and vermin that can cause endemic typhus, plague, rat-bite fever, and food infections. Through food substances, man may get flukes from freshwater snails, crabs, and fish; tapeworms and other parasites from meat; intestinal disorders from food contaminated by insects; and tularemia and Rocky Mountain spotted fever from wild game.

Before an agent can cause any damage to the body it must gain entry. These portals of entry include the skin surfaces, the respiratory tract, the gastrointestinal tract, and the genitourinary tract. Most infections gain entry through the mouth in food and water and from the fingers and other objects that are placed in the mouth. Whooping cough, influenza, the common cold, and tuberculosis are transferred through the air and enter the body through the nose as we breath. Both the nose and mouth are gateways to the respiratory and digestive tracts. The genitourinary tract is a portal of entry for microorganisms of venereal disease, trichomoniasis, and yeast infections. The skin is a common portal of entry because of the large number of pathogens to which it is exposed. If the skin is intact, most of the biologic agents cannot cross this barrier.

*Clostridium tetani*, the cause of tetanus, is a normal inhabitant of soils and is found in the intestinal tract of wild and domesticated animals and is rarely found in man. *C. tetani* gains access into subsurface tissue via punctures, lacerations, and contusions. The infection is called *lockjaw* because of the painful spasms that occur in the muscles of the jaw and neck. The jaws may become immovable in severe and terminal cases. The incubation varies from 2 to 50 days but is usually 4 to 14 days. Immunization against tetanus has contributed to a decreased incidence of the disease.

*Clostridium botulinum* causes food poisoning. This is a result of ingestion of toxic-contaminated food, with only a small amount being required to cause severe symptoms and even death. Botulism in human beings almost always results from eating improperly preserved, canned, or processed foods. Botulinus toxins can be produced in foods that are not obviously spoiled. These toxins can be inactivated by boiling food for 10 to 15 min.

*Neisseria gonorrhoeae* is the etiologic agent of gonorrhea. It is the most common and widespread of all the venereal diseases and is worldwide in distribution. The organism is transmitted by sexual intercourse but can be transmitted to an infant by contact with an infectious discharge from the mother during birth. This may lead to blindness if unattended.

The gonococcus causes an infection of mucous membranes, chiefly of the genitourinary tract. The organism penetrates between the surface epithelium, setting up an inflammatory infection in the subepithelial tissue that becomes purulent. In males the infection spreads to the urethra, prostate gland, and epididymis. Symptoms are a burning sensation in the urethra and on urination and a purulent exudate at the urethral orifice. Sterility may result from destruction of the epididymis by the inflammatory process. In the female the infection spreads to the urethra, vagina, cervix, and fallopian tubes. The first symptoms are an irritating discharge, burning on urination, and swelling of the Bartholin glands. Sometimes there may be little discomfort, so that she may be unaware that she is infected.

Typhoid fever is a communicable disease caused by *Salmonella typhosa*. It is usually acquired by the ingestion of food or water contaminated with urine or feces of infected persons. The incubation period is usually 10 to 14 days, during which time the organisms have penetrated the intestinal mucosa and entered the lymphatic vessels and mesenteric nodes. Onset is characterized by malaise, anorexia, and headache. A severe fever develops and is accompanied by prostration, nosebleeds, either diarrhea or constipation, rose spots, intestinal bleeding, and occasionally perforation of the bowels.

Laboratory diagnosis of *Salmonella* infections is accomplished by isolation by culture of the organism. It is also useful to demonstrate a rise in antibody titer during the course of the disease.

Staphylococci (grapelike cocci) cause a number of diseases. These include furuncle (boil), carbuncle, acne, impetigo, abscess, osteomyelitis, arthritis, tonsillitis, sinusitis, otitis media, bronchitis, acute enteritis, food poisoning, bacteremia, and septicemia.

*Staphylococcus aureus*, a gram-positive coccus, is the most common cause of pyogenic infections, such as of the skin, subcutaneous tissues, and wounds. Impetigo is a contagious infection found in children, involving the superficial layers of the skin with pustules, vesicles, crusts, and bullae. It is a typical abscess formation that is usually localized. The carbuncle is a more complex focal lesion extending deep into the tissue with suppurative pockets and is usually found on the back of the neck.

*Staphylococcus* food poisoning is probably the most common type of food poisoning. The symptoms occur rapidly and are of short duration. The usual symptoms are nausea, vomiting, severe abdominal cramps, and diarrhea.

Some 50% to 60% of the population are carriers of pathogenic staphylococci, particularly in the anterior nares. Almost all carry the nonpathogenic *S. epider-*

*midis* on the skin. Therefore these carriers continuously transfer staphylococci to susceptible individuals. Hospital epidemics are not uncommon in nurseries and surgical wards.

Streptococci infections (90%) are caused by *Streptococcus pyogenes*. Whereas infections caused by staphylococci produce a thick, purulent discharge, infections caused by streptococci produce a thin, watery discharge. The focal lesions produced are otitis media, appendicitis, impetigo, wound infections, tonsillitis, and pharyngitis. The more generalized diseases include puerperal sepsis, bronchopneumonia, meningitis, erysipelas, scarlet fever, and septicemia.

*Streptococcus viridans* (alpha or nonhemolytic) is found in the nose and throat of normal individuals and is a normal inhabitant of the small intestine. *S. pyogenes* (beta hemolytic) is the cause of sore throat or nasopharyngitis. It may remain localized or may spread to other areas.

Erysipelas is a diffusely spreading infection. It usually involves the subcutaneous tissue of the face, but the trunk or extremities may be involved. The lesions are marked by a fiery red discoloration and edema.

Scarlet fever begins with severe pharyngitis, tonsillitis, vomiting, and headache. Erythrogenic toxin is produced and causes typical erythematosus manifestations. The Dick test is performed to reveal susceptibility or immunity to scarlet fever.

Nonsuppurative diseases of serious consequence may develop as a sequelae to a not-so-serious initial streptococcal infection. Rheumatic fever and acute hemorrhagic glomerulonephritis are examples. Although the exact pathogenesis of rheumatic fever is not known, it seems to be the result of a series of immunologic reactions instituted by serial infections with almost any group A streptococci. Acute glomerulonephritis is a complication caused by a limited number of strains. It is believed that the streptococci activate the autoimmune mechanism that causes formation of antibodies to the kidney.

The predominant disease caused by *Streptococcus pneumoniae* is a lobar-type pneumonia. In addition to the involvement of the lungs, the paranasal sinuses and middle ear are often sites of infection. Meningitis in both adults and children is often the result of pneumococcal infections as well as empyema, lung abscess, purulent pericarditis, acute bacterial endocarditis, and myocarditis.

Meningococcal meningitis is caused by *Neisseria meningitidis*. The source of infection is often a healthy carrier or someone who has recently recovered from the infection. The bacteria enter the body through the nose and mouth and are spread by droplets in the air following sneezing and coughing or by direct contact. The disease begins wtih local nasopharyngeal infection, sudden severe headache, and stiffness and pain in the neck, shoulders, and back. The fever is high, and nausea and vomiting often occur. Symptoms may progress to delirium, stupor, or even coma. Without treatment it is fatal in about half of the cases.

## THROAT CULTURE

PRINCIPLE: Throat cultures are important as aids in the diagnosis of certain infections such as streptococcal sore throat and diphtheria; in establishing the focus of infection in diseases such as scarlet fever, rheumatic fever, and acute hemorrhagic glomerulonephritis; and also in the detection of the carrier state of

**63**

organisms such as beta hemolytic streptococci, meningococci, *S. aureus*, and diphtheria bacilli.

REAGENTS:

1. Blood agar: Add 5% to 10% sterile defibrinated blood to melted nutrient agar that has been cooled to about 45° C.
2. Chocolate agar: nutrient agar is cooled to 75° C, and 10% sterile defibrinated blood is added and mixed.

PROCEDURE:

1. Depress patient's tongue and rub swab firmly over back of his throat. Care should be taken to avoid touching tongue or lips with swab.
2. Inoculate a blood agar and a chocolate agar plate.
3. Streak both plates for isolation.
4. Place in a 37° C incubator.
5. Observe in 24 hours.

INTERPRETATION: The following organisms are considered normal flora:

| | |
|---|---|
| Alpha hemolytic streptococci | Pneumococci |
| *Neisseria catarrhalis* | Nonhemolytic streptococci |
| *Staphylococcus epidermidis* | Diphtheroid bacilli |
| *Haemophilus influenzae* | |

The following organisms are considered pathogenic:

| | |
|---|---|
| Beta hemolytic streptococci | *Bordetella pertussis* |
| *Corynebacterium diphtheriae* | Meningococcus |

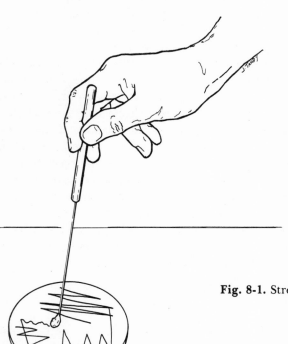

**Fig. 8-1.** Streaking for isolation.

64

If there is a predominance of *Staphylococcus aureus*, coliform bacilli, pneumococci, *H. influenzae*, and *Candida albicans,* it is considered pathogenic.

## STAINING OF BACTERIA

PRINCIPLE: Bacteria are minute, almost colorless cells invisible to the naked eye. Unstained bacteria are difficult to observe even with the aid of a microscope. To make them more easily observable, bacteria may be stained with dyes. Before being stained, bacteria are suspended in a drop of water on a clean microscope slide and then spread in a thin, even film. The film is allowed to air dry, and the organisms are "fixed" to the slide by gentle heat or by chemical means. The preparation is known as a fixed smear, which is then stained.

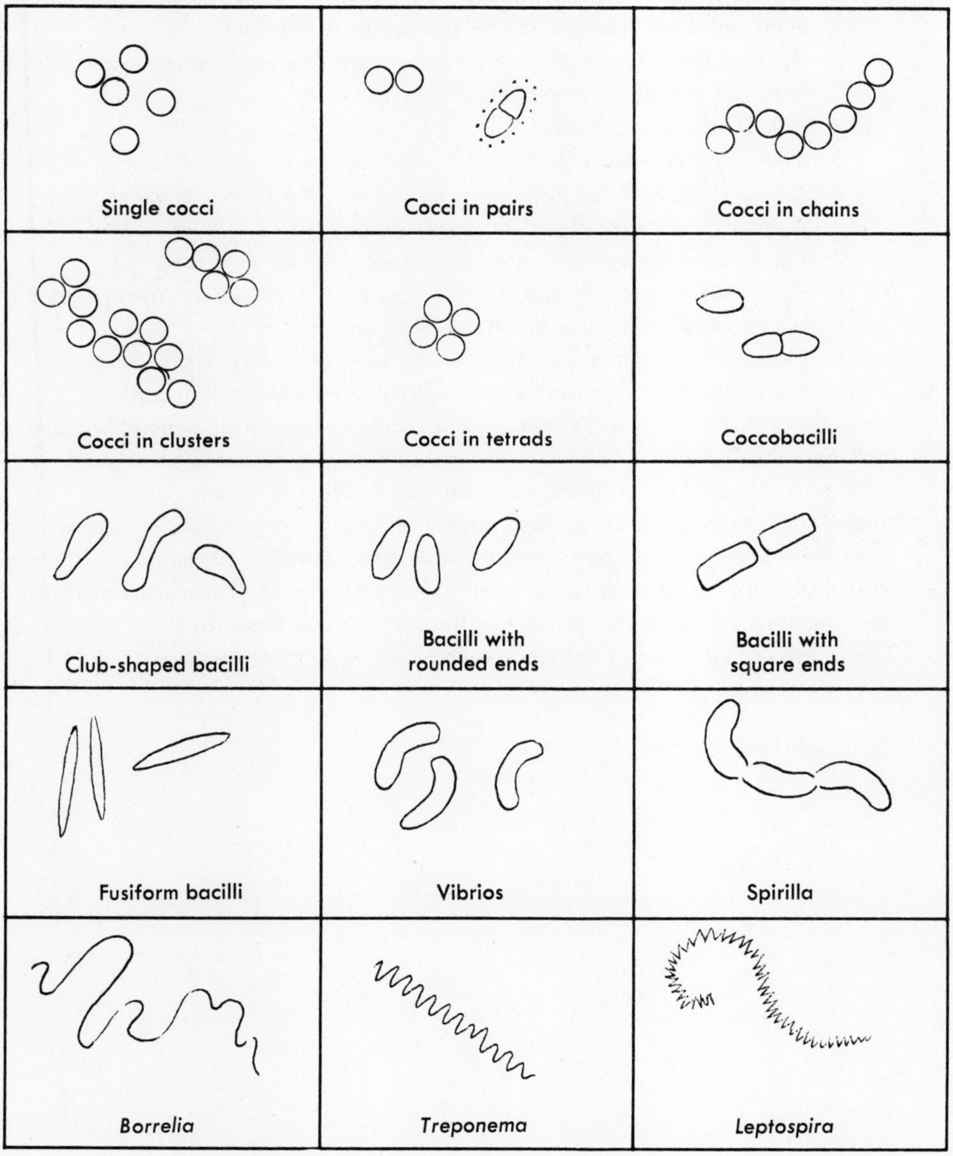

**Fig. 8-2.** Morphology of bacteria.

1. Crystal violet 0.5% in distilled water
2. Gram's iodine:
   1 g iodine
   2 g potassium iodide
   300 ml distilled water
3. Acetone
4. Safranin 0.5% in distilled water

PROCEDURE:

1. On a clean slide place a loopful of water.
2. Transfer a very small amount of bacteria from one of the colonies you have selected using a sterile inoculating needle.
3. Spread bacteria over an area about the size of a dime to get a thin film. Sterilize needle immediately after making smear.
4. Allow slides to air dry.
5. Pass slide through flame, film side up, two or three times.
6. Cover slide with crystal violet, letting it remain 15 sec. Wash stain off with a gently flowing stream of tap water.
7. Cover with iodine solution for 30 sec. Wash with water.
8. Cover with acetone, agitate slide gently for 10 sec or until no more color is removed from smear. Wash with water.
9. Counterstain with safranin for 30 sec, and wash with water.
10. Carefully blot dry and examine using oil immersion lens.

INTERPRETATION: Gram's stain is a differential staining procedure discovered by Christian Gram in 1884 when he was staining bacteria in tissues. It is very useful in the differentiation of bacteria, especially those that have the same shape and size but differ in their ability to retain a crystal violet–iodine complex when washed with a decolorizer (acetone). Microorganisms that retain the complex and remain violet are called gram positive. Microorganisms that give up the complex and become colorless when washed with acetone are gram negative. These microorganisms take up a second stain or counterstain.

*See worksheet, p. 115.*

# 9 Serology

## SEROLOGIC REACTIONS

The combination of antigen with antibody is the basic reaction behind most immunologic procedures. This reaction is relatively specific (able to discriminate between antigens of similar structure). If an antigen-antibody complex precipitates, the antibody is called a *precipitin*. If the antigen is a toxin, the antibody that neutralizes it is an *antitoxin*. If the antigen is on the cell surface and reaction with the antibody causes the cells to agglutinate, the antibody is called an *agglutinin*. When cell lysis occurs, the antibody is a *lysin*, and if it renders the cell susceptible to phagocytosis, it is an *opsonin*.

Serologic tests may be used in several different ways to identify the causative agent in a variety of disease states. Even after clinical manifestations of a disease have disappeared, antibody production may continue. The presence of an elevated antibody titer to an organism indicates that infection has occurred at some time. An etiologic agent may be identified and a diagnosis established by testing serum with a variety of antigens from different suspected microorganisms.

The most frequently used serologic test is that for syphilis. Syphilis is an infection caused by the spirochete *Treponema pallidum*. This is the most important venereal disease because of its devastating systemic effects. Syphilis is contracted through sexual intercourse, but the infection may be transmitted through blood transfusion, and an infected mother can pass the infection to offspring in utero.

During the first stage of syphilis a chancre appears on the genital organs. This occurs from 10 to 30 days after contact with an infected person. This chancre is hard and varies from a small erosion to a deep ulcer. It usually occurs on the vulva in females and on the urethra in males. Chancres may also occur on the fingers, lips, and elsewhere on the body. These chancres heal within 4 to 6 weeks.

The secondary stage begins about 2 to 10 weeks after the appearance of the chancre. The symptoms include malaise, generalized lymphadenopathy, and a papular eruption occurring in the mouth, vulva, vagina, and rectum. The lesions will subside spontaneously within a few weeks, but if untreated, the lesions reoccur for several months to 3 years. This is when the spirochetes enter the bloodstream.

The tertiary stage may not appear for 8 to 25 years after the initial infection. All tissues and organs may be involved in this stage. Most severely affected are the cardiovascular system, central nervous system, skeletal system, skin, and upper respiratory tract. Syphilitic aortitis is one of the most common lesions. It has also been responsible for pathologic reactions in the central nervous system and is responsible for about 33,000 patients in mental institutions in the United States. In the central nervous system it occurs as meningovascular syphilis and paresis (general paralysis of the insane). Intracranial nerves may be damaged, causing deafness and visual disturbances.

Syphilis cannot be diagnosed solely on clinical manifestations, since it is a great mimic of many diseases. The diagnosis depends on demonstration of organisms and specific antibodies. The tests most often employed are the VDRL (Venereal Disease Research Laboratory), the RPR (rapid plasmin reagin), and the TPI (*Treponema pallidum* immobilization).

## RPR TEST FOR SYPHILIS

PRINCIPLE: The RPR card test utilizes carbon particles coated with cardiolipin as the antigen. Many body tissues contain cardiolipin. One theory why cardiolipin reacts in the nontreponemal tests for syphilis is that the treponema itself has an antigenic marker closely related to cardiolipin, and therefore the treponema stimulates antibody against cardiolipin. Another theory, and the more popular of the two, is that the treponema invading the tissues releases cardiolipin from hidden sites in the body cells and tissues, and this newly revealed cardiolipin stimulates the antibody-forming mechanism.

REAGENTS: Available as a kit from Hynson, Westcott and Dunning, Inc.

PROCEDURE:

NOTE: Controls, RPR card antigen suspension, and test specimens should be at room temperature when used.
1. Squeeze Dispenstir near stirring or sealed end and draw up serum sample.
2. Hold Dispenstir directly over card area and allow 1 drop to free fall onto card.
3. Invert Dispenstir, and with sealed stirring end, spread specimen in confines of circle.
4. Shake antigen dispensing bottle before use. Holding in a vertical position, dispense one free-falling drop on each test area. Do not restir.
5. Rotate for 8 min under humidifying cover on mechanical rotator at 100 rpm. Or if hand method is used, rock and tilt card slowly (approximately 20 to-and-fro motions per minute) for a maximum of 4 min.

INTERPRETATION: Report as reactive or nonreactive.
1. Reactive: showing characteristic clumping ranging from slight but definite to marked and intense.
2. Nonreactive: showing slight roughness or no clumping.

Biologic false-positive reactions are sometimes caused by diseases such as infectious mononucleosis, leprosy, SLE, vaccinia, and viral pneumonia. The extent to which these affect the RPR test has not been completely determined, but they have been known to affect other nontreponemal tests for syphilis and should be considered when running an RPR.

## RHEUMATOID ARTHRITIS TEST

PRINCIPLE: Serum from patients with rheumatoid arthritis contains a factor that can be used for differential diagnosis. This rheumatoid factor is a protein of molecular weight between 900,000 and 950,000 belonging to the IgM class. Rheumatoid factor is regarded as an autoantibody against antigen determinants of IgG.

The principle of the test is an immunologic reaction between rheumatoid factors (antibody) and the corresponding antigen, which is heat-denatured human IgG coated on the surface of biologically inert latex particles. The rheumatoid factor differs from normal IgM in that it will react to heat-denatured IgG.

REAGENTS: Available as a kit from Wampole Laboratories, Dist.

PROCEDURE:

1. Place 1 drop of patient's serum on one section of glass slide.
2. On another section of slide, place 1 drop of positive control.
3. Add 1 drop eosin reagent to patient and control drops. Stir mixture in each section with clean stirrer.
4. Add 2 drops latex reagent to patient and control drops. Again stir mixture in each section with clean stirrer, spreading over an area of about 2.5 sq cm (1 sq in).
5. Rock slide gently for 3 min and immediately observe for agglutination.

INTERPRETATION: Report as

1. Negative: a homogeneous red suspension without visible agglutination.
2. Weak positive: agglutination visible, but particles are small and develop slowly. Clumping may be incomplete.
3. Strong positive: extensive agglutination; large particles that appear very quickly; pattern comparable to that seen in the positive control.

The rheumatoid arthritis test is often positive in patients with SLE, syphilis, and in some cases of hepatic disease. Rheumatic fever gives a negative reaction.

## PREGNANCY TESTING

PRINCIPLE: Human chorionic gonadotropin (HCG) appears in the urine of pregnant females, and determination of its presence generally indicates a positive test for pregnancy.

Utilizing an immunologic technique based on the principle of indirect agglutination, tests will detect HCG at levels of 1.5 to 2.5 International Units (IU) per milliliter. Since levels as low as 1.5 IU have been reported as early as 5 days after the first missed period, negative tests should be repeated within 1 to 2 weeks.

Test components consist of an antigen in the form of suspension of HCG chemically bonded to latex polymer particles and an antiserum containing antibodies to HCG. When the antiserum is mixed with urine containing a detectable level of HCG, it is neutralized, and no agglutination occurs. This is a positive test for pregnancy. Urine that contains no HCG cannot neutralize the antiserum, resulting in agglutination of the latex reagent. This indicates a negative test for pregnancy.

**69**

Patients with chorioepithelioma or hydatid mole frequently excrete HCG in the urine. Therefore a positive result obtained when testing these patients does not always indicate a positive test for pregnancy.

REAGENTS: Available as a kit from Roche Diagnostics.

PROCEDURE:

1. Drop 1 drop urine in circle on glass slide.
2. Add 1 drop antiserum reagent.
3. Stir and rotate gently for 30 sec.
4. Add 1 drop antigen reagent.
5. Mix over entire circle.
6. Rotate slide vigorously for no longer than 2 min while observing for agglutination.

INTERPRETATION: Report as

1. Positive test: No agglutination within 2 min. HCG present in the urine of pregnant women will inhibit agglutination of latex particles in the antigen reagent, resulting in a smooth, milky appearance after rotation.
2. Negative test: Any degree of agglutination within 2 min. Lack of HCG in the urine of nonpregnant women permits agglutination of the antigen and antiserum reagents within a 2 min period, producing easily recognizable clumping of the latex particles.

*See worksheet, p. 117.*

# Worksheets

NAME _____

DATE _____

Choose the word or words in column B which describe the prefix, stem, or suffix listed in column A.

| Column A | Column B |
|---|---|
| _____ epi- | a. eye |
| _____ endo- | b. liver |
| _____ osteo- | c. intestine |
| _____ myo- | d. wall of a structure |
| _____ arthro- | e. blood |
| _____ phlebo- | f. ear |
| _____ oto- | g. within, inside |
| _____ -emia | h. kidney |
| _____ mono- | i. muscle |
| _____ myelo- | j. bone |
| _____ nephro- | k. vein |
| _____ hemo- | l. joint |
| _____ hepato- | m. spinal cord |
| _____ arterio- | n. on, upon |
| _____ ren- | o. below or low |
| _____ hypo- | p. artery |
| _____ hyper- | q. mouth |
| _____ entero- | r. skin |
| _____ encephalo- | s. midline |
| _____ stoma- | t. around |
| | u. brain |
| | v. posterior |
| | w. above or high |
| | x. one |

Fill in the blank with the letter of the correct statement.

1. _____ The term intravenous means
   a. Around a vein
   b. Within a vein
   c. Beneath a vein

73

2. _____ Extracellular means
   a. Within a cell
   b. Beneath a cell
   c. Outside a cell

3. _____ Subcutaneous means
   a. Adjacent to the skin
   b. Beneath the skin
   c. Within the skin

4. _____ Which of the following terms means between the ribs?
   a. Intracostal
   b. Infracostal
   c. Intercostal

5. _____ Post mortem means
   a. Before death
   b. After death
   c. Causing death

6. _____ Monomorphic means having which form or shape?
   a. A single form or shape
   b. Many forms or shapes
   c. An unusual form or shape

7. _____ A person suffering from a disease characterized by polyuria would void
   a. Urine tinged with blood
   b. A small amount of urine
   c. A large quantity of urine

8. _____ Hypertension refers to
   a. Elevated blood pressure
   b. Low blood pressure
   c. Absence of blood pressure

9. _____ The condition characterized by a rapid heart beat is called
   a. Bradycardia
   b. Arrhythmia
   c. Tachycardia

10. _____ In the term bradycardia, the prefix *brady-* means
   a. Sporadic
   b. Slow
   c. Rapid

Fill in the blank with the appropriate word or words.

1. Leukocyte refers to a _____ blood cell.

2. Erythrocyte refers to a _____ blood cell.

3. Cyanosis refers to the condition of being _____ in color.

4. The word anteroposterior would be translated as from _____ to back.

5. Dysuria describes _____ urination.

74

6. Nocturia refers to a condition characterized by excessive urination during the _____.

7. Lymphadenopathy refers to a disease of the lymph _____.

8. Arthritis refers to an inflammation of a _____.

9. Pneumonitis refers to inflammation of the _____.

10. The term myocardium refers to the _____ muscle.

11. Hepatitis refers to an infection which is centered in the _____.

12. The term hematuria refers to _____ in the urine.

13. Lipoma refers to a tumor which is composed of _____ tissue.

14. Cholelithiasis describes a disease state characterized by the presence of gall _____.

15. Neuritis describes inflammation of a _____.

16. Phlebitis refers to inflammation of a _____.

17. The term hepatoma describes a _____ of the liver.

18. Leukopenia is a blood disorder characterized by too _____ leukocytes.

19. Inflammation of the stomach is known as _____.

20. Hyperglycemia refers to _____ sugar in the blood.

21. Nephritis means inflammation of the _____.

22. The excision of part of the intestine is known as an _____.

23. A word that refers to inflammation of the heart is _____.

24. A word meaning inflammation of bones is _____.

25. The adjective meaning above the pelvis is _____.

26. Tachycardia means _____ _____ _____.

27. _____ means a temporary cessation of breathing.

28. The study of blood is _____.

NAME _____

DATE _____

Unknown No. _____

    Hematocrit _____

    Hemoglobin _____

    White blood cell count _____

Your results:

    Hematocrit _____

    Hemoglobin _____

NAME _____

DATE _____

Write a brief definition to each of the following terms.

1. Anisocytosis _____

_____

2. Band cell _____

_____

3. Basophilic _____

_____

4. Eosinophilic _____

_____

5. Erythrocyte _____

_____

6. Hypochromic _____

_____

7. Microcyte _____

_____

8. Normochromic _____

_____

9. Poikilocytosis _____

_____

10. Polychromatophilia _____

_____

11. Reticulocyte _____

_____

12. Thrombocyte _____

_____

NAME _____

DATE _____

Your results:

| | | Normal adult differential ranges: | |
|---|---|---|---|
| Neutrophilic band cells | _____% | Neutrophilic band cells | 2% to 6% |
| Neutrophils | _____% | Neutrophils | 50% to 70% |
| Lymphocytes | _____% | Lymphocytes | 25% to 40% |
| Monocytes | _____% | Monocytes | 3% to 8% |
| Eosinophils | _____% | Eosinophils | 1% to 4% |
| Basophils | _____% | Basophils | 0% to 1% |

NAME _____

DATE _____

Record results and make interpretation on the following chart concerning your own blood type.

Cell reaction with anti-sera

| Anti-A | Anti-B | Anti-A,B | Anti-Rh$_0$(D) | Albumin control |
|--------|--------|----------|----------------|-----------------|
|        |        |          |                |                 |

Cells are group        _____

Cells are Rh        _____

Unknown sample No. _____

Reverse grouping

| Anti-A | Anti-B | Anti-A,B | A cells | B cells | Anti-Rh$_0$(D) | Albumin control |
|--------|--------|----------|---------|---------|----------------|-----------------|
|        |        |          |         |         |                |                 |

Cells are group _____

Cells are Rh        _____

Reverse grouping interpretation (group _____)

NAME _____

DATE _____

Given the following reactions, fill in the ABO types on patients 1 to 8.

| Grouping | ABO type | Anti-A | Anti-B | A cells | B cells |
|---|---|---|---|---|---|
| Forward | | | | | |
| Patient 1 | _____ | + | − | Not tested | Not tested |
| Patient 2 | _____ | + | + | Not tested | Not tested |
| Patient 3 | _____ | − | + | Not tested | Not tested |
| Patient 4 | _____ | − | − | Not tested | Not tested |
| Reverse | | | | | |
| Patient 5 | _____ | Not tested | Not tested | + | + |
| Patient 6 | _____ | Not tested | Not tested | − | + |
| Patient 7 | _____ | Not tested | Not tested | − | − |
| Patient 8 | _____ | Not tested | Not tested | + | − |

NAME _____

DATE _____

Direct antiglobulin

    Unknown No. _____

    Results _____

    Unknown No. _____

    Results _____

Indirect antiglobulin

    Unknown No. _____

    Results

| Screening cells | Immediate spin | Albumin 37° C | AHG |
|---|---|---|---|
| I | | | |
| II | | | |

NAME _____

DATE _____

Give brief definitions for the following.

1. Acute _____
   _____

2. Agglutination _____
   _____

3. Agglutinin _____
   _____

4. Agglutinogen _____
   _____

5. Anamnestic response _____
   _____

6. Anaphylaxis _____
   _____

7. Anemia _____
   _____

8. Antibody _____
   _____

9. Antigen _____
   _____

10. Bilirubin _____
    _____

11. Coated cells _____
    _____

12. Complement _____
    _____

13. Fetal _____
    _____

14. Globulin _____
    _____

15. Hemoglobin _____

_____

16. Hemolysis _____

_____

17. Immunized _____

_____

18. Infusion _____

_____

19. Inter- _____

_____

20. Intra- _____

_____

21. Intravenously _____

_____

22. Jaundice _____

_____

23. Landsteiner's rule _____

_____

24. Maternal _____

_____

25. Normal saline _____

_____

26. Plasma _____

_____

27. Reagent _____

_____

28. Red blood cells _____

_____

29. Sensitivity _____

_____

30. Serum _____

_____

31. Specificity _____

_____

32. Transfusion _____

_____

NAME _____

DATE _____

Capillary resistance test          _____ petechiae

Bleeding time (Duke method)    _____ min

Results of buccal smear _____

How many Barr bodies were in each nucleus? _____

NAME _____

DATE _____

## URINALYSIS

Physical analysis

    Color _____

    Transparency _____

    Specific gravity _____

Chemical analysis

    pH _____

    Albumin _____

    Glucose _____

    Ketone bodies _____

    Occult blood _____

    Bilirubin _____

    Urobilinogen _____

    Other _____

Microscopic examination (high power field)

    WBC _____

    RBC _____

    Epithelial cells _____

Casts (low power field)

    Hyaline _____

    Fine granular _____

    Coarse granular _____

    Mucous threads _____

    Bacteria _____

    Crystals _____

Technologist _____

Date and time collected _____ Date completed _____

NAME _____

DATE _____

## CALCULI ANALYSIS

Source _____

Weight _____ Consistency _____

Chemical analysis

    Ammonium _____    Phosphates _____

    Calcium _____    Urates or

    Carbonates _____      uric acid _____

    Cystine _____    Other _____

    Magnesium _____    Category of stone _____

    Oxalate _____

Technologist _____

Date and time collected _____ Date completed _____

1. A Fahrenheit thermometer reads 59°. What would be the comparable centigrade temperature?

2. Convert a Fahrenheit temperature reading of 302° to a centigrade reading.

3. Convert a centigrade thermometer reading of 60° to a Fahrenheit reading.

4. What does a centigrade reading of −23° equal on the absolute scale?

5. How many grams of $NaCl$ are needed to make 1 liter of a 2 M solution?

6. What weight of $NaCl$ is needed to make 1 liter of a 0.2 M solution?

7. How many grams of potassium nitrate ($KNO_3$) are needed to make 1 liter of a 1.0 N solution?

8. To make 500 ml of a 0.1 N solution of calcium ($CaCl_2$), how many grams of the salt are required?

9. How would you make 1 liter of a 0.04 N solution from a 0.8 N solution?

10. How many milliliters of 0.1 N $NaOH$ will 10 ml of 1 N hydrochloric acid ($HCl$) neutralize?

11. Five ml of urine is diluted to 100 ml, and 1 ml of this solution is diluted 1:10. What is the final concentration of urine in the solution?

NAME _____

DATE _____


Control _____ mg/dl

Unknown _____ mg/dl

NAME _____

DATE _____

Control _____ mg/dl

Unknown _____ mg/dl

NAME _____

DATE _____

Control _____ mg/dl

Unknown _____ mg/dl

NAME _____

DATE _____


Control _____ mg/dl
Unknown _____ mg/dl

Serum thymol turbidity

    Control    _____ units

    Unknown _____ units

Serum total bilirubin

    Control    _____ mg/dl

    Unknown _____ mg/dl

**Toxicology**
(pp. 55-57)

NAME _____

DATE _____

Acid-neutral extract _____

Alkaline extract        _____

NAME _____

DATE _____


Control  _____ mg/dl

Unknown _____ mg/dl

NAME _____

DATE _____

Results of throat culture

    Macroscopic description of colonies:

      Blood agar _____

_____

      Chocolate agar _____

_____

    Microscopic description of colonies:

      Gram stain _____

_____

      Morphology _____

_____

NAME _____

DATE _____

Rapid plasmin reagin

No. _____   _____

No. _____   _____

Rheumatoid arthritis

No. _____   _____

Control        _____

Pregnancy testing

No. _____   _____

# Index

**119**